Essentials of Rheumatology

WE 540 C11   Fanfare 12631
          25/7/85   4.95

Essentials
of Rheumatology

H L F Currey
Professor of Rheumatology
and Director of the
Bone and Joint Research Unit,
The London Hospital Medical College
Honorary Consultant Rheumatologist,
The London Hospital

Pitman

PITMAN BOOKS LIMITED
128 Long Acre, London, WC2E 9AN

PITMAN PUBLISHING INC.
1020 Plain Street, Marshfield, Massachusetts

Associated Companies
Pitman Publishing Pty Ltd, Melbourne
Pitman Publishing New Zealand Ltd, Wellington
Copp Clark Pitman, Toronto

First published 1983

Library of Congress Cataloging in Publication Data

Currey, H L F
  Essentials of rheumatology.
  Includes index.
  1. Rheumatism. I. Title. [DNLM: 1. Rheumatology—Handbooks. WE 140 C976e]
RC927.C86   616.7′23   82–7487
ISBN 0–272–79677–8   AACR2

British Library Cataloguing in Publication Data

Currey, H L F
  Essentials of rheumatology.
  1. Rheumatism
  I. Title
  616.7′23   RC927

ISBN 0 272 79677 8

Text set in 10/12 pt Linotron 202 Times, printed and bound in Great Britain at The Pitman Press, Bath

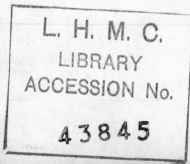

Contents

This table of contents is arranged to provide a simple classification (or at least a check-list) of rheumatological conditions.

Preface

When asked what reading material they want for studying rheumatology our medical students are surprisingly consistent in their replies:

a concise systematic text
short enough for rapid revision
well indexed
small enough for the pocket of a white coat
inexpensive

This is an attempt to fill these requirements.

I believe that medical students are not alone in needing such a text. Today's physiotherapists, occupational therapists and nurses dealing with rheumatic diseases also require a concise account of clinical rheumatology. I hope this will meet their needs too.

The text can be read straight through as a systematic account of the subject—or it can be dipped into, starting either from the index (which has been prepared with particular care) or from the table of contents, which is set out in the form of a classification of rheumatic diseases. All classifications have shortcomings, but I believe that students find it helpful to have some framework which indicates the whole content of the subject. The inclusion of a page reference for each condition in this classification should allow the reader to move straight to the relevant page in the text.

Unlike reviewers of books for undergraduates, students themselves, in my experience, do not favour literature references. These have therefore been omitted. I have not excluded brief mention of rarities: part of the value of a book such as this is as a dictionary to look up unfamiliar terms. I have attempted to provide very full cross referencing within the text. This avoids repetition and, I hope, will help the reader.

I have been exercised as how best to make the text suitable for use in rapid revision. Insertion of bold tabular material has advantages, but breaks up the text. I have therefore made extensive use of italics to highlight key words within the text. I hope that this, combined with use of page references in the classification (table of contents) will facilitate revision.

1 Structure and Function of Joints

Figure 1.1 shows the structure of a typical synovial joint. Additional 'spacers' may be present in the form of fibrocartilage (e.g. knee menisci) or fat pads covered by synovium.

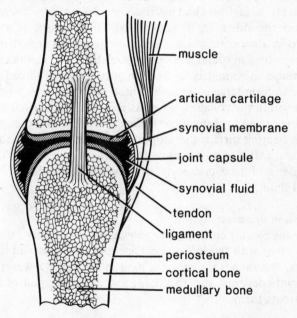

Figure 1.1 Diagram of a normal synovial joint. A muscle acting across the joint has been included to emphasise the important function of such muscles in maintaining joint stability

The structure of intervertebral joints is considered on page 68 (Fig 7.1).

Synovium
The folded synovial lining consists of 1 to 2 layers of cells of two types: phagocytic 'A' cells which are involved in clearing material from the joint, and synthetic 'B' cells which produce protein and hyaluronate. This layer lies on vascular subsynovial connective tissue.

Synovial fluid

The normal joint contains only a small volume of synovial fluid (clinical evidence of fluid always indicates an abnormality). The fluid is viscous due to about 2 per cent *hyaluronate*.

The synovial fluid lubricates the bearing surfaces, the *protein* content being essential for this. In addition, the fluid acts as the vehicle for transporting nutrients to the cartilage, and wear/waste products to the 'A' lining cells for removal by phagocytosis.

Articular (hyaline) cartilage

Like other connective tissues, hyaline cartilage consists of three components: cells, fibres and matrix. The cells are *chondrocytes*; they synthesise the other components. The fibres consist of *collagen*, arranged in a network which binds the cartilage to underlying bone and sweeps up and round in loops through the 1 to 3 mm thickness of the cartilage. The matrix consists of *proteoglycans* linked to hyaluronate to form large *aggregates*. These long, coiled aggregates are trapped within the collagen network. Because proteoglycans absorb water, they swell to distend the collagen network and thus give this cartilage bearing surface the properties of a firm elastic cushion.

Articular cartilage possesses neither nerves nor blood vessels. It is insensitive, and the chondrocytes are nourished by diffusion from the synovial fluid.

Capsule and ligaments

The fibrous *capsule* encloses the synovial tissues. It resists distension and, together with the inelastic collagenous *ligaments* and the bony contours, determines the range of joint movement. However, *stability* of joints depends also to a large extent on the pull of muscles acting across them.

Joint sensation and pain

Synovial tissues are poorly innervated, but the fibrous structures—capsule, ligaments and periosteum—have a rich sensory supply. These tissues are probably the main source of pain in arthritis. With advanced joint damage deep bone sensation is probably also involved.

2 Rheumatoid Arthritis

Rheumatoid arthritis (RA) is the most common and serious type of inflammatory polyarthritis. The inflammation affects primarily synovium and may lead to severe joint destruction. Although the brunt of the disease falls on the joints, it is a systemic condition and, together with disorders such as SLE, ranks as a *systemic connective tissue disease* (p 32).

Epidemiology

RA affects about 2 per cent of the population, more commonly females (3:1). The peak age of onset is in the fifth decade, but it may start at any age (in children merging into chronic juvenile arthritis— p 15). Slight familial clustering occurs, and a modest increase in HLA-DR4 points to a genetic influence.

Aetiology, pathogenesis and serology

The cause is unknown. A central event appears to be the formation of *immune complexes* within the joint. These activate *complement* and attract *neutrophils*. Phagocytosis of immune complexes by neutrophils releases chemical mediators of inflammation. Continued inflammation stimulates the synovium to proliferate as granulation tissue (*pannus*) which erodes cartilage and bone. Extra-articular lesions may represent systemic immune complex deposition. Characteristically the serum contains *rheumatoid factors*—autoantibodies directed against IgG (i.e. antiglobulins or anti-antibodies—*see* p 132). Although not specific for RA, being found for example in some cases of liver disease, these rheumatoid factors are valuable diagnostic markers. They are probably an important constituent of the pathological immune complexes.

The underlying cause remains an enigma. The immunological activity points to a provoking antigen, which might be a virus, an altered 'self' component, or possibly IgG. The genetic link with HLA-D locus genes suggests that predisposition may depend on a particular state of immune reactivity.

3

Pathology

Synovium. The synovial lining cells multiply to become several layers deep and the surface is thrown into finger-like villi. *Fibrin* is deposited on the surface.

The subsynovial tissues are infiltrated with *plasma cells* and *lymphocytes*, the latter often arranged as *follicles*, occasionally with paler *germinal centres*. These appearances come to resemble an immunologically active lymph node. Immunofluorescent staining shows many of the plasma cells to be synthesising *rheumatoid factors*. Very few neutrophils are seen in the synovium (in contrast to the large numbers in the synovial fluid—p 135).

As inflammation continues outgrowths of vascular granulation tissue—*pannus*—spread from the synovial margin across the cartilage to invade through cartilage into the bone ends, producing *erosions*. Other changes include increased vascularity, oedema and fibrosis.

The above description refers to the fully developed situation. Two important points must be noted. Firstly, in the early stages (when diagnostic biopsy is likely to be performed) the synovial changes may be very insignificant. Secondly, even the fully developed picture is non-specific. With the possible exception of immunochemical staining tests, similar changes may be seen in the seronegative spondarthropathies (p 19) such as ankylosing spondylitis, and occasionally in SLE (p 33).

Tendon sheath synovial linings undergo inflammatory changes similar to those of the joint synovium.

Subcutaneous nodules. These highly characteristic lesions consist of a central core of *fibrinoid necrosis* surrounded by a radiating *palisade of epithelioid cells* (macrophages). Outside this are *lymphocytes* and *plasma cells*.

Arteries. Vascular involvement probably underlies most of the extra-articular features. Arterial changes range from bland intimal hyperplasia (giving nail-fold lesions—p 7) to vessel wall necrosis of the type seen in polyarteritis nodosa (p 43) in rare, severe cases.

Clinical features

Joints
A characteristic onset of RA is the appearance of a *symmetrical small joint polyarthritis* affecting the hands and feet, and associated with

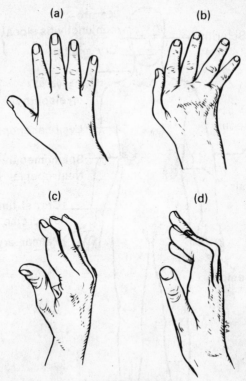

Figure 2.1 Typical rheumatoid hand deformities
(a) Early fusiform swelling of proximal interphalangeal finger joints.
(b) Ulnar deviation of fingers (with metacarpophalangeal subluxation.
(c) Swan neck finger deformities
(d) Boutonnière finger deformities

early morning stiffness. Raynaud's phenomenon (p 40 and *carpal tunnel syndrome* (p 105 may be premonitory symptoms. Before long, *fusiform swellings* of the PIP joints give the fingers a spindled appearance (Fig 2.1), and the patient is unable to make a fist (like carpal tunnel compression this may point to early tendon sheath swelling). Irritable MTP joints may produce a sensation that the balls of the feet are treading on marbles. *Morning stiffness*—lasting up to some hours—becomes a prominent and distressing symptom. Affected joints are tender, with thickened synovium and effusions.

Less often the onset is *monarticular, episodic* (palindromic—p 113) or even *extra-articular*. There may be some systemic disturbance, but the onset is usually dominated by joint pain, morning stiffness—and anxiety.

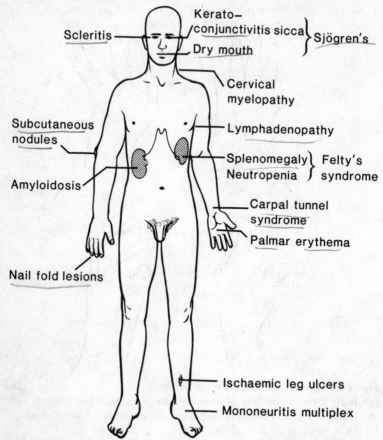

Figure 2.2 Some of the extra-articular manifestations of rheumatoid arthritis

With progression of the disease there may be spread to almost every joint in the body. The *wrists* are often severely affected, and their involvement is a diagnostic pointer to inflammatory arthritis as opposed to osteoarthritis, in which they are spared. In the *spine* only the *upper cervical* region is usually involved, probably because of the numerous synovial articulations there.

More advanced disease may produce flexion deformities, subluxation and instability (aggravated by muscle wasting). Characteristic hand changes include *MCP subluxation*, *ulnar deviation* of fingers, *boutonnière* and *swan-neck* deformities (Fig 2.1). Flexion and varus deformities of the knee are the commonest cause for taking to a wheelchair.

Joint damage in the *upper cervical spine* may produce *spinal cord damage* either through loss of the transverse ligament of the atlas allowing this vertebra to slip forward on the axis, or subluxation at C2–C5 levels. Lateral X-rays in flexion are needed to demonstrate this. *Note the grave dangers of manipulating the rheumatoid cervical spine*.

Carpal tunnel syndrome (p 105) may occur at any stage of RA. It is easily treated, but failure to detect it may allow serious functional deterioration by adding a neurological defect to a hand already compromised by articular and tendon sheath problems.

Synovial rupture of the knee (p 115) may mimic deep vein thrombosis.

Extra-articular features (Fig 2.2)

Weight loss, low grade *fever* and *lymph node enlargement* are features of active disease.

Subcutaneous nodules are painless, shotty lumps $\frac{1}{2}$ to 3 cm in diameter found typically over the olecranon, but sometimes over other bony prominences or arising from tendons, particularly the tendo Achilles. They occur only in those with positive tests for rheumatoid factor and, apart from occasional patients with SLE (p 33), are diagnostic of RA.

Tendon sheaths and bursae are lined with synovium and may become inflamed and distended by fluid. This is most commonly recognised in the wrist and hand. Apart from palpable swellings, tendon sheath involvement can cause *trigger finger* (p 106), *ruptured tendons* or *carpal tunnel syndrome* (p 105).

Arteritis is a marker of severe disease. In the fingers it produces 'nail-fold lesions': brown/black skin infarcts 1 to 2 mm in diameter. Larger vessel involvement may produce *leg ulceration* or a type of peripheral neuropathy due to occlusion of vasa nervorum: *mononeuritis multiplex*. This occurs as a phase of severe systemic rheumatoid disease. The stepwise evolution of the neuropathy—one peripheral nerve being picked off after another over a period of days or weeks—is highly characteristic and is similar to that seen in polyarteritis nodosa (p 44), which condition this form of RA may come to resemble: '*malignant rheumatoid*' (an example of overlap between the systemic connective tissue diseases—p 33.

The lungs may be affected by *fibrosing alveolitis* or *nodules* which develop in the parenchyma, and sometimes cavitate. When pneumoconiosis affects a seropositive rheumatoid patient this tends to produce large dense peripheral opacities on X-ray (*Caplan's syndrome*).

Pleural effusion, usually unilateral, affects particularly men. The sterile fluid characteristically has a low glucose content (less than 1.5 nmol/l).

The eye may be involved in various ways. Up to 30 per cent of all rheumatoid patients have *Sjögren's syndrome* (*Kerato-conjunctivitis sicca*—p 56), while a few severe, long-standing cases develop *scleritis*: episodes of scleral inflammation which leave tell-tale areas of bluish pigmentation. Rarely this progresses to *scleromalacia perforans* from rupture of a scleral nodule.

Heart lesions are seldom recognised in life. At post-mortem there may be evidence of *pericarditis* or *myocardial nodules*. Rarely *endocarditis* produces mitral or aortic valve murmurs.

NSAID

Anaemia is common. It is most often due either to the influence on the marrow of *chronic inflammation* or to *iron deficiency* secondary to insidious gastrointestinal bleeding caused by analgesics. The differentiation between these may be difficult. Both may produce microcytosis with low serum iron values. However, the total iron binding capacity (TIBC) is low with chronic inflammation, high with iron deficiency. As a rule a favourable response to iron therapy can be expected if the TIBC is greater than 55 μmol/l the serum ferritin less than 55 μg/l. The absence of stainable iron in a marrow smear is more direct evidence of iron deficiency.

Felty's syndrome is an uncommon development in which *neutropenia* and *splenomegaly* appear, usually late in the course of RA. Severe neutropenia may lead to infections. *Thrombocytopenia, haemolytic anaemia, skin pigmentation*, and *leg ulceration* are occasional features. The mechanism of the neutropenia is unknown.

The course of Felty's syndrome is unpredictable. If recurrent infections become a problem or the neutrophil count falls to dangerous levels, both *corticosteroids* and *splenectomy* may produce a remission, but this is sometimes temporary, and the condition can be fatal.

Less common extra-articular manifestations include *cutaneous vasculitis, myopathy* and *symmetrical (glove-and-stocking) peripheral neuropathy*.

Investigations

Blood picture
The *ESR* provides a convenient index of inflammatory activity. *Anaemia* (p 8) and *thrombocytosis* are common.

Tests for rheumatoid factor
The actual tests are described in Appendix B (p 132). The *latex test* (positive ≥1/80) is a simple routine test positive in 80 per cent of RA patients. The various *sheep cell agglutination tests* (positive ≥1/16) are more specific but less sensitive. In most cases of RA the tests become clearly positive early on and remain positive. More severe diseases and particularly extra-articular features are associated with higher titres of rheumatoid factors. These tests are of fundamental importance in the diagnosis of RA. However, some cases of otherwise typical RA remain seronegative throughout, while a few normal people have positive tests.

Antinuclear antibodies
About 20 per cent of RA patients, particularly women, have positive *ANA* or *LE cell tests* (p 133). The DNA binding test (p 133) is however negative. This serological overlap can produce difficulties in differential diagnosis.

Radiology
A common error is to order too many X-rays. The progress of erosive changes can be followed on two standard films: one showing both hands and wrists, the other both feet. Other sites should be X-rayed only to answer specific questions. The radiological changes in RA and osteoarthritis are contrasted in Table 6.1 and Figure 6.1 (pp 66 and 65). The changes of RA include:

Soft tissue swelling such as the spindle-shaped outline of fingers due to PIP joint swelling.

Periarticular osteoporosis, which contrasts with the bone sclerosis seen in osteoarthritis (p 63.)

Eorsions of the bone cortex (Fig 6.1). These are holes in the periarticular bone which open on to the surface (in contrast to the cysts of osteoarthritis—p 63). They are the radiological hallmark of the 'inflammatory' arthropathies (i.e. RA and the seronegative group).

Narrowing of the joint space is a non-specific sign of joint damage due to loss of the (radiolucent) articular cartilage 'spacer'.

Periosteal reaction may be apparent as a faint line of periosteal new bone formation along the shafts of bones adjacent to affected joints, particularly in children.

Later deformities include destruction of bone ends and subluxation.

Diagnosis

Fully developed RA is unmistakable, with symmetrical polyarthritis, morning stiffness, raised ESR, positive latex and sheep-cell tests, radiological erosions and subcutaneous nodules. However, problems arise with the early, incomplete case. Thus the onset may be monarticular, palindromic (p 113) or polymyalgic (p 45). Further, there may be confusing overlap (both clinical and serological) with other systemic connective tissue diseases (p 32). The combination of erosions and positive rheumatoid factor tests almost invariably signifies RA. Nodules clinch it. Synovial histology can place the condition in the 'inflammatory polyarthritis' group (and exclude conditions such as tuberculosis) but cannot specifically identify RA. Some cases can be labelled only 'possible' or 'probable' RA until the condition evolves more completely.

Complications

Amyloidosis is discovered (usually unexpectedly) in about 15 per cent of autopsies on patients with longstanding RA. Occasionally it presents clinically, particularly as proteinuria. *Rectal biopsy* is a convenient screening test.

Septic arthritis is a rare but definite complication of RA. Thus an undue exacerbation in a rheumatoid joint is an indication for diagnostic aspiration.

Prognosis

Disease activity waxes and wanes spontaneously. Of those patients referred to hospital with RA, about half will either go into remission or run a mild course without developing serious disability. The remainder develop progressive disease which leads to more or less incapacity. About 10 per cent finish in wheelchairs. Females generally fare less well than males, but serious extra-articular disease is more common in men. High titres of rheumatoid factor and the presence of nodules and other extra-articular features indicate a worse prognosis.

Death directly attributable to RA is uncommon but may result from cervical subluxation (p 7), amyloidosis (p. 10), arteritis (p 7), Felty's syndrome (p 8) or from complications of treatment.

Treatment

No prevention or cures are available but much can be done to improve the lot of the patient with RA. Management strategy includes, firstly, measures directed at the patient and the disease (drugs and surgery etc.) and, secondly, modification of the activities and environment to overcome functional problems.

Rest

Contrary to traditional views, rest is not of proven value in RA. Nevertheless, during phases of excessive inflammatory activity, a period of bed rest and/or splinting of the most active joints may give some relief.

Physiotherapy, occupational therapy, etc.

Exercises play a fundamentally important part in management. Active exercises against resistance are the only effective means of strengthening muscles acting across diseased joints, thus improving *stability* and *range of movement*.

Warming or cooling the joint can provide temporary pain relief (as a hot-water bottle will relieve abdominal pain) and this may make exercises easier to perform. It is however important to appreciate that electrical gadgetry is only a means to more effective exercising. Short-wave diathermy etc. are of no proven therapeutic value on their own.

The remedial services provide many other facilities for the rheumatoid patient, including selection and instruction in the use of *walking aids, footwear, modifications in the home*, and *gadgets* etc. In addition they design and make *splints*, the purpose of which may be to rest a joint, to provide stability at a joint while a limb is in use or to prevent or correct a joint deformity.

Drugs

Analgesic/anti-inflammatory agents. RA is a painful, inflammatory disease, and most patients require regular medication with full doses of one or two drugs which have both anti-inflammatory and analgesic properties. These drugs can be expected to reduce pain, shorten early morning stiffness and lessen joint swelling. They do not alter the course of the disease. They are referred to as *non-steroidal anti-inflammatory drugs* (NSAID). All inhibit the synthesis of prostaglandins, but it is uncertain to what extent this action accounts for their effectiveness—or their gastric irritant properties.

Soluble aspirin (900 mg qid), because of gastric intolerance, is now less favoured that the newer preparations. A typical starting regimen is naproxen 250 mg tid plus indomethacin 75 mg on retiring. Individual patients vary in their acceptance of particular NSAID. Other preparations which can be tried include benorylate suspension (10 ml bd), ibuprofen (400 mg tid), ketoprofen (50–100 mg bd), flurbiprofen (50 mg tid), fenoprofen (600 mg tid), diclofenac (50 mg tid), sulindac (100–200 mg bd), tolectin (300 mg tid) and piroxicam (20 mg once daily).

Simple analgesics. It is helpful to provide an additional analgesic for use when needed (unlike the above NSAID which should be maintained in regular full doses). Drugs used in this way include *paracetamol, codeine, 'Distalgesic'*, and *diflunisal*.

Slow-acting ('suppressive') drugs. Drugs such as gold lack analgesic and conventional anti-inflammatory (aspirin-like) properties, but bring about a gradual reduction in disease activity over a period of months. All are potentially very toxic and are used only when RA is severe and progressive. Strict monitoring is needed. This group includes the drugs shown in Table 2.1. They are given concurrently with analgesic/anti-inflammatory agents. At present penicillamine and gold are used more than the immunosuppressives (because of the small but definite risk of malignancy) and hydroxychloroquine, which is probably less effective. An oral gold preparation ('Auranofin') is at present being tested.

penicillamine

Table 2.1 Slow acting drugs used in RA

Drug	Dosage	Major toxicity	Monitoring
Gold (sodium aurothiomalate)	(im injection) Test dose 10 mg, then 50 mg weekly to 1g, then 50 mg monthly	Bone marrow suppression Skin rash Nephropathy Stomatitis	Enquire: rash/pruritis Urinalysis monthly Blood count monthly*
Penicillamine	125 mg daily increasing by monthly steps to 500–750 mg/daily	Bone marrow suppression Nephropathy Skin rash Taste loss Various other syndromes	Blood count 2–4 weekly* Urinalysis 2–4 weekly General interrogation
Immunosuppressives Azathioprine	2.5 mg/kg/day	Bone marrow suppression Teratogenesis Oncogenesis Sterility	Blood count monthly*
Cyclophosphamide	1.5 mg/kg/day	Cyclophosphamide: cystitis alopecia	Cyclophosphamide: urinalysis monthly
Chlorambucil	0.5 mg/kg/day		
Hydroxychloroquine	200 mg daily (maximum 2 years)	Retinopathy	Specialist ophthalmic monitoring

* Including differential and platelet counts.

Corticosteroids are the only drugs which dramatically suppress rheumatoid inflammation. Unfortunately their cumulative side effects make their use justifiable only in exceptional circumstances. Intolerable pain and disability (despite other drugs) occasionally force their use. Prednisolone is the preparation of choice, keeping the dose if possible to 7.5 mg daily or lower. More than 10 mg daily places the patient on a collision course.

Rarely, large doses are needed to tide a patient over a phase of severe systemic involvement (p 7).

Local injections of corticosteroids (e.g. hydrocortisone acetate 100 mg for a knee joint) may be useful for suppressing a flare in a single joint. The effect lasts only days or weeks. Intra-articular radioisotopes (e.g. Yttrium^{90}) are being evaluated as a means of ablating the active rheumatoid synovium.

Surgery
A variety of operations can dramatically improve rheumatoid joints, but there is a limit to what should be undertaken in the individual patient with progressive polyarthritis. The ideal subject for surgery is the patient in whom one particular joint is causing a major problem. In these circumstances *total replacement* of a hip, knee or finger joints can be highly effective. *Excision arthroplasties* for painful metatarsophalangeal joints, and *fusion* of unstable wrist joints are other useful procedures. A wide variety of other operations, such as cervical fusion, nerve entrapment releases or ankle stabilisation may be required for particular problems. Surgical synovectomy of rheumatoid joints produces short-term pain relief, but the long-term effects are uncertain.

3 Juvenile chronic arthritis

When diseases such as rheumatoid arthritis and ankylosing spondylitis affect children, the manifestations differ from those in the adult. It is not clear to what extent childhood arthropathies should be regarded as the equivalents of adult conditions. What is clear is that grouping together of all childhood inflammatory arthropathies as *'Still's disease'* or *'juvenile rheumatoid arthritis'* is an over-simplification. A number of different conditions are involved. At present these are most usefully classified according to the pattern of clinical presentation. Collectively they are called *juvenile chronic arthritis (JCA), defined as arthritis starting below the age of 16 and affecting four or more joints for at least three months, or fewer joints for this period with biopsy confirmation, other diseases being excluded.*

JCA is rare. Occasionally the childhood clinical picture may first appear later in life ('adult Still's disease'). No more is known about the aetiology and pathogenesis of JCA than is discussed under the adult inflammatory arthropathies (pp 3, 19).

Clinical types

Systemic
This presents as a systemic illness with high swinging fever worse in the evenings and associated with a fleeting macular rash. Other features include lymphadenopathy, hepatosplenomegaly, pericarditis and pleurisy. The onset is usually between the ages of 1 to 3 years. Arthritis may not appear until weeks or months after the onset. The severity varies. Often it resolves, but about a quarter of patients develop progressive and destructive arthritis. Iridocyclitis does not occur. Tests for rheumatoid factors and antinuclear antibody (ANA) are negative.

Polyarticular, rheumatoid factor negative
Most common in younger girls, this type may develop mild systemic features. Only 10 to 15 per cent develop serious joint destruction.

Polyarticular, rheumatoid factor positive

Affecting mainly older girls, this type often comes to resemble adult rheumatoid arthritis. It can produce progressive joint damage. Subcutaneous nodules often occur. ANA is positive in 75 per cent.

Pauci-articular arthritis

There are two subgroups in whom only a few joints (six or less) are involved:

(a) Usually affects girls under the age of five. Extra-articular manifestations are uncommon except for *chronic iridocyclitis* which affects about 50 per cent—particularly those with *positive antinuclear antibody tests*. The arthritis usually resolves, but the insidious iridocyclitis may lead to blindness. *Regular (three-monthly) ophthalmological screening is mandatory*. Rheumatoid factor tests are usually negative.

(b) Usually affects older boys. Lower limb large joint involvement tends to be followed by sacroilitis and spondylitis. It is often associated with HLA-B27 and probably represents a juvenile form of ankylosing spondylitis. *Iridocyclitis* may occur, but presents as an acute, red painful eye. Tests for ANA and rheumatoid factors are negative.

Other types

Rarely, children may develop chronic arthritis in association with psoriasis, inflammatory bowel disease or one of the other systemic connective tissue diseases (p 32).

Clinical and radiographic features

Some of the clinical features are mentioned above. In young children it may take considerable experience to detect arthritis. *Bony joint fusion* is more common than in adult rheumatoid arthritis. It may affect particularly the wrist and neck.

The relatively thick articular cartilage in children means that bony erosions develop late. *Sub-periosteal new bone formation* characteristically appears in relationship to inflamed joints. Bone growth is also affected, and in individual bones may be either retarded or accelerated. A late result of this may be a *hypoplastic mandible* (receding chin) or *shortening of a metacarpal or metatarsal*. The cervical spine may show *fused and underdeveloped vertebrae*. There may also be general *stunting of growth* (apart from stunting induced by steroid treatment).

Fever tends to be intermittent, and may be high. The *rash* consists of pale macules which are evanescent, appearing during febrile periods. *Hepatosplenomegaly* and *lymphadenopathy* sometimes occur.

Investigations

Raised ESR and anaemia reflect disease activity. A marked *neutrophil leucocytosis* may occur. Plasma globulins are elevated and, as mentioned above, some children have positive tests for rheumatoid factor and/or antinuclear antibodies.

Diagnosis

In the systemic type it may initially be very difficult to tell whether the child has a rheumatic disorder. Once it is apparent that the child has arthritis, it is necessary to consider *rheumatic fever* (p 97). (The arthritis is 'flitting' and the ASO test indicates a recent streptococcal infection.) *Infections* have to be excluded, particularly if a single joint is involved. If suspected, synovial fluid (if necessary a biopsy specimen of synovial membrane) must be obtained for microbiological examination. A variety of *viral infections*, including rubella (p 95) may cause a subacute self-limiting polyarthritis. *Acute leukaemia* can closely mimic polyarthritis. Bone marrow examination may be needed to exclude it.

Prognosis

The various types of JCA carry differing prognoses. In general, children's joints fare better than those of adults with comparable involvement. Complicating *amyloid disease* may be fatal, and insidious iridocyclitis, if undetected, may lead to blindness.

Management

The more severe cases of JCA require expert management and extensive resources if their psychological and educational development is to be maintained while their painful inflammatory disease is controlled, and contractures and deformities prevented. Active disease may require bed rest and splinting of joints as well as individual physiotherapy and other measures. Drug therapy is broadly similar to that employed for adult rheumatoid arthritis (p 12). *Gold* (starting dose 0.5 to 1 mg/kg body weight weekly), *penicillamine* and *hydroxy-chloroquine* can all be employed, but immunosuppressives are seldom felt to be justified unless the child develops amyloidosis. *Corticosteroids* are generally avoided because of cumulative side effects. In children stunting of growth is a particular hazard. There is some evidence that alternate daily steroid dosage may reduce some side effects. One clear indication for steroids is iridocyclitis to prevent blindness.

Surgery is a more difficult proposition in children than in adults because the epiphyses are open and the bones growing. Most of the operative procedures carried out in the adult (p 14) are occasionally performed in children, but the long-term results are less well known.

4 Seronegative spondarthritis (and 'reactive arthritis')

The classification of conditions described in this chapter is difficult. The various disorders are closely linked genetically and pathologically, and exhibit considerable clinical overlap. Yet this inter-relationship is not understood, nor is it clear exactly which diseases fall within the group (some include Whipple's disease—p 116, and Behçet's syndrome—p 109). Four relatively well defined conditions are generally accepted as constituting the group:

Ankylosing spondylitis
Psoriatic arthritis
Reiter's disease
Enteropathic arthritis

The awkward title 'seronegative spondarthritis' reflects the fact that these disorders were originally separated from rheumatoid arthritis because they all lack serum rheumatoid factors (pp 9, 132). However, 'seronegative arthritis' would be an insufficient title, for a few cases of what appear to be typical rheumatoid arthritis are also seronegative (p 9). The term 'spondarthritis' indicates the central position of spondylitis in the overlapping clinical network within the group.

These conditions tend to cluster together in families—often different disorders within the same family—and this clustering is largely explained by association with *HLA-B27*.

The use of tissue typing has made necessary some changes in the concept of seronegative spondarthritides. For example, the anterior uveitis and aortitis which sometimes complicate ankylosing spondylitis or Reiter's disease may occur in HLA-B27 subjects as isolated features, without any joint disease. Some argue that the various clinical features—spondylitis, peripheral arthritis, skin lesions, aortitis, uveitis etc.—may appear in isolation or in any combination, depending on the interplay of genes, particularly HLA-B27. This concept of *HLA-B27-related diseases* may be valid. However, at a clinical level it remains helpful to consider the conditions as if they are separate entities (which is what is done in this chapter) while recognising the overlap between them.

Discussion of seronegative spondarthritis requires consideration also of the concept of '*reactive arthritis*'. This term has been used to describe a sequence suspected of taking place for example in Reiter's disease, in which an infection in the genitourinary tract or bowel triggers off a polyarthritis which is independent of the original infection. The polyarthritis which may follow *Yersinia enterocolitica* infections (p 91) is probably similarly 'reactive' and, intriguingly, these patients also show an association with HLA-B27. The question therefore arises whether the common factor in the seronegative spondarthritides may be a genetically determined tendency to develop reactive arthritis. This is somewhat implied by describing (venereal) Reiter's disease as *sexually acquired reactive arthritis* ('SARA'). In fact, 'reactive arthritis' at present remains an interesting concept rather than a diagnosis, and the triggering mechanism has not yet been proved to be a factor common to all the seronegative arthritides. Other arthritides with 'reactive' features are rheumatic fever (p 97) and certain cases of gonococcal arthritis (p 93).

The association between HLA-B27 and the seronegative arthritides, particularly ankylosing spondylitis, remains unexplained. One hypothesis suggests that a nearby gene on chromosome 6 determines a particular state of immune reactivity, another postulates that the B27 antigen in the cell membrane bears antigenic resemblances to certain infecting organisms. This might result either in foreign organisms being treated as 'self' antigens or reactions against foreign organisms cross-reacting against normal tissues.

Ankylosing spondylitis

Ankylosing spondylitis (AS) is a form of seronegative spondarthritis involving particularly the spine and affecting mainly young adult males. Bony ankylosis is a feature of severe cases. Ninety per cent of patients possess HLA-B27 (compared with an overall 8 per cent in white populations). Some B27-positive people who do not satisfy the criteria for classical AS may nevertheless suffer minor aches on this account.

Aetiology

The association with HLA-B27, and the presence of AS in 3 per cent of first degree relatives points to a strong genetic factor. Further, overlap with Reiter's disease, and the association of B27 and 'reactive arthritis' (p 20) suggest that AS could also represent a 'reactive arthritis'. This remains a possibility which is being intensively investigated, but so far no infective or other 'trigger' has been identified.

Prevalence, sex and age of onset

In White populations about 0.1 per cent suffer from classical AS. It is suspected that in a larger number of people HLA-B27 is associated with less specific aches. Classical AS affects 5 men to 1 woman. If mild disease is included the sex difference is less marked (sex may influence severity rather than frequency of AS). The age of onset is most commonly between 17 and 25, but it can start at any age. AS almost never occurs in pure black populations (which lack HLA-B27).

Associated conditions

Patients suffering from AS may exhibit a variety of related conditions, including *peripheral arthritis* (35 per cent), *episodic acute anterior uveitis (iritis)* (30 per cent), *psoriasis* (5 per cent), *ulcerative colitis* or *Crohn's disease* (5 per cent), *aortic incompetence* or *cardiac conduction defects* (3 per cent). These associated disorders behave neither like complications of AS, nor like 'trigger' factors precipitating AS. Rather it is as if they are independent conditions occurring in the same individual.

Clinical features

The first symptom is typically *low backache* which extends to the buttocks and thighs. This is often worse at night and associated with *morning stiffness*. Later the pains extend up to the thoracic cage and neck. Although usually insidious, the onset may occasionally be acute and mimic a lumbar disc lesion. Sometimes one of the associated conditions mentioned above may appear before the spondylitis.

In the early stages examination may reveal some restriction of lumbar spine motility (in all directions, in contrast to the usual limitation only of flexion in disc lesions), and tenderness and pain on stressing the sacroiliac joints (p 126). It is possible that minor expressions of AS are common in those with HLA-B27, and that many never even reach the stage of seeking medical advice.

Not all the skeletal symptoms arise from joints. Spondylitic patients tend to develop periosteal reactions with laying down of new bone at sites of tendon and ligament insertions (*enthesopathy*).

This may present as *painful heels* (plantar fasciitis—p 107, or 'Achilles' tendinitis—p 106), or *pain and tenderness over the iliac crest or ischial tuberosity*.

In those patients in whom AS progresses, the process appears to involve first the sacroiliac joints, then spreads upwards to affect progressively the lumbar, dorsal and thoracic segments of the spine. Initially the pain and stiffness are due to inflammation, and both can be reversed by anti-inflammatory drugs plus exercises (a useful diagnostic point). Later true *bony ankylosis* can supervene, with *spinal rigidity* which is not reversible by drugs. The final picture may be that of a rigid 'poker spine'. At this stage pains may be less troublesome, but lack of cervical rotation is a handicap. Spinal rigidity is paralleled by rib cage immobility due to costovertebral joint involvement. *Chest expansion* often falls below the lower normal limit of about 5 cm.

Uncomplicated ankylosing spondylitis usually does not prevent the patient continuing his work. However, severe disability may result either from gross spinal flexion deformity or from peripheral joint disease. Severe *flexion deformities* are now becoming rare, due, it is thought, to the modern practice of treatment by exercise and avoidance of immobility (*see under* Treatment). *Peripheral arthritis* occurs in 30 per cent. This is somewhat similar to rheumatoid arthritis, but is predominantly lower limb and tends to spare the hands and wrists. *Hip joint involvement* is a particular hazard. It is especially disabling in a patient whose spine is rigid.

Associated conditions

A number of conditions may co-exist with ankylosing spondylitis. As explained on page 21, these appear neither to act as aetiological 'triggers', nor to represent complications of the ankylosing spondylitis. Rather, they appear to be independent, separate disorders. They include:

Iritis (acute anterior uveitis). Thirty per cent of ankylosing spondylitis patients experience attacks of acute, usually unilateral, iritis. The painful, red eye responds well to corticosteroids.

Heart disease. About 1 per cent of patients develop inflammation of the proximal aorta, resulting in aortic valve incompetence. Less common lesions include conduction defects, cardiomyopathy and pericarditis.

Inflammatory bowel disease. Either ulcerative colitis or Crohn's disease occurs in 5 per cent of patients with ankylosing spondylitis. In contrast to enteropathic arthritis (p 31) the colitis and arthritis fluctuate independently. In addition, when patients with ankylosing spondylitis who do not complain of bowel symptoms are screened by endoscopy etc., a larger proportion shows some evidence of unsuspected large bowel inflammation.

Reiter's syndrome (p 28) and *reactive arthritis* (p 20) may both be associated with spondylitis features, occasionally with fully developed ankylosing spondylitis.

Complications

Spinal fractures may occur, despite buttressing by new bone formation, because the spine is rigid and porotic.

Amyloidosis occurs, but is rare.

Pulmonary problems are less common than might be expected in a disease which may severely restrict thoracic breathing, presumably because diaphragmatic breathing is maintained. Very rarely *apical pulmonary fibrosis* may occur and mimic tuberculosis.

Painful heel (p 107) or *Achilles tendinitis* sometimes occur, and may be early features.

Romanus lesions are relatively uncommon inflammatory lesions affecting the edge of one or more vertebrae adjacent to the disc. They are often painful. Radiographically they appear as erosive defects which may closely mimic an infective lesion.

Investigations

The *sedimentation rate* is generally raised in proportion to the inflammatory activity, but unexpectedly high or low readings also occur. Tests for *rheumatoid factor* are negative, but about 85 per cent of patients possess *HLA-B27*.

X-ray changes are characteristic in advanced cases. The sacroiliac joints are irregular, with sclerotic edges and erosions, or bony fusion. The characteristic late spinal change is bony bridging between adjacent vertebrae by *syndesmophytes* and bony fusion of facetal joints, producing eventually a solid, rigid bony tube, the *bamboo spine* (Fig 7.2, p. 70). The normal concavity of the vertical borders of the vertebral bodies may give way to a *squared* appearance, while *Romanus lesions* (p 23) are occasionally seen. Bony prominences such as the heel may show fluffy new bone growth.

Diagnosis

The fully developed disease with a 'poker spine' is unmistakable, although the possible associations listed on page 22 need also to be considered.

Until recently it was believed that radiological sacroiliitis was an almost invariable accompaniment of ankylosing spondylitis. However, it now appears that patients possessing HLA-B27 may present with rather vague low backache or a picture which resembles a disc lesion, but without clinical or radiological evidence of sacroiliitis.

Ankylosing spondylitis needs to be considered in all patients presenting with backache or more diffuse skeletal pains. Pointers to inflammatory spondylitis in such cases include a past history of iritis, painful heel, or a family history of any seronegative spondarthritis or one of the associated conditions mentioned on page 21. Particularly significant is a history of morning stiffness (lasting more than 30 minutes) with diffuse pains which extend to the chest, and buttocks. A dramatic response to drugs such as indomethacin, or a favourable influence of physical activity (as opposed to rest) may have been noted. Physical examination sometimes reveals tenderness over the sacroiliac joints (the site is marked by a pair of skin dimples) or there may be limitation of *lateral* bending of the lumbar spine.

The ESR is a valuable screening test, but can be misleadingly normal. Radiological sacroiliitis is the most valuable confirmatory test (the other X-ray changes are relatively late). A standard view of the pelvis is usually sufficient for assessing the sacroiliac joints. However, below the age of 18 years the appearance of the immature joints is almost impossible to interpret. Obviously, irradiation particularly of the pelvis is undesirable in young people. *Do not order unnecessary X-rays*.

Tissue typing is at present an expensive test in short supply. Its use should be limited to patients who present diagnostic problems and in whom management will be influenced by the result of the test.

Prognosis

At one end of the scale the classical disease may progress to a rigid, poker spine which, although uncomfortably awkward and somewhat disfiguring, generally allows the patient to continue at work. At the other end of the scale, depending on the criteria for diagnosis, is probably a considerably larger number of people who have much milder manifestations, and some of whom probably never even consult a doctor.

Correct management almost certainly improves the prognosis for pain, motility and posture. The 'doubled-up' flexion deformity of the older textbooks appears to be avoidable.

Associated conditions (p 22), particularly hip involvement, or complications (p 23) may become a greater problem than the spondylitis.

Treatment

The cornerstone of management is a combination of an anti-inflammatory drug and active physical exercise.

Anti-inflammatory drugs are much more effective than in rheumatoid arthritis. Phenylbutazone (100 mg tid) was for long the drug of choice but, because of the slight risk of bone marrow suppression, indomethacin (25 mg tid) is now widely used. Most of the newer anti-inflammatory drugs (e.g. Piroxicam 20 mg each morning) are also proving effective, so there is a wide choice. After an initial response the dose is titrated down to the minimum which will maintain comfort.

Active exercise is at least as important as drugs. A discipline of regular (daily) physical activity such as swimming, cycling, walking or physical jerks is required. Some like to follow a planned physiotherapy routine. The choice is determined by what produces the best patient compliance. This is one disease in which rest is positively harmful. If a patient with ankylosing spondylitis is confined to bed for any reason (such as an operation) it is important to arrange physiotherapy in bed.

X-ray therapy was at one time widely used. Irradiation of the spine can produce improvement comparable to that achieved by anti-inflammatory drugs. However, like the latter it probably does not influence the long-term outcome. It has fallen from favour because it increases the risk of leukaemia by a factor of 10 times, and also because of the availability of effective drugs. It is still occasionally used, in doses up to 1,500 rad, for those in whom anti-inflammatory drugs fail for any reason. It is ineffective for peripheral joint involvement.

Peripheral joint involvement is managed along lines similar to rheumatoid arthritis, except that slow-acting drugs (and corticosteroids) are avoided. The tendency to bone overgrowth may shorten the effective functioning life of prosthetic hip joint replacements.

Iritis requires prompt treatment with a mydriatic and topical steroids.

Avoidance of spinal trauma is advisable because the porotic and rigid spine is liable to fracture. Car seat headrests should be used, and recreations such as skiing avoided.

Psoriatic arthritis

This is a form of 'seronegative spondarthritis' (p 19) in which psoriasis is associated with polyarthritis somewhat resembling rheumatoid arthritis, but tending to be less symmetrical and to involve terminal interphalangeal joints and the spine.

Incidence and aetiology

and no subcutaneous nodules.

Psoriatic arthritis is about five times less common than ankylosing spondylitis. It affects adults of any age and is slightly more common in women. There is some familial clustering. It occasionally first appears in childhood. There is considerable clinical overlap with other forms of 'seronegative spondarthritis' (p 19) and it is notable that histology of the skin lesions in Reiter's disease is similar to that of cutaneous psoriasis. Aetiology is considered further on p 20.

Clinical features

Polyarthritis often presents like rheumatoid arthritis (p 3), and differentiation between the two conditions may be difficult. Features which favour psoriatic arthritis include a more *episodic, asymmetrical pattern* of joint involvement. One or a few finger joints may be involved in acute, destructive episodes. A characteristic feature is arthritis of *terminal interphalangeal joints* of fingers, often with the nail on the same finger being distorted by psoriatic involvement (pitting, 'ladder pattern' or subungual hyperkeratosis) or involvement of *interphalangeal toe joints*. The bulbous swellings of terminal interphalangeal joints have to be differentiated from Heberden's nodes (p 64) and gouty tophi (p 83). Cervical spine involvement is common. There may also be sacroilitis and other features of spondy-litis, ranging up to full-blown ankylosing spondylitis. Those with spondylitis are more likely to possess HLA-B27 (p 19). In general the arthritis tends to be milder and less destructive than rheumatoid. However, the occasional case of psoriatic arthritis progresses to very severe destructive changes ('arthritis mutilans'), with loss of bone ends in digits, resulting in shortened, telescoping fingers ('main en lorgnette'). In the fingers or toes a combination of interphalangeal joint and flexor tendon sheath swelling may produce the character-istic appearance of 'sausage digits'.

Skin lesions are usually present before arthritis appears, and there may be a family history of psoriasis. Occasionally it may be difficult to detect the psoriasis, especially if lesions are limited for example to the finger nails, scalp, natal cleft or umbilicus. Exceptionally the arthritis actually precedes the skin lesions, in which case a tentative diagnosis may, nevertheless, be possible on the basis of the pattern of joint involvement.

Investigations

The sedimentation rate and ESR parallel inflammatory activity as in rheumatoid arthritis. X-rays also show similar changes, except that the destructive finger joint lesions produce osteolysis: the bone ends taper down and disappear. There may be evidence of sacroiliitis and spondylitis. Amongst those patients with spondylitis (but not those without), about 60 per cent possess HLA-B27. Tests for rheumatoid factor are negative. Synovial histology is similar to the rheumatoid joint. Extensive psoriasis may produce a modest elevation in plasma uric acid, presumably through the increased rate of cell turnover.

Diagnosis

Problems arise in differentiating psoriatic arthritis from rheumatoid arthritis, and also in labelling cases which exhibit overlap with the other seronegative spondarthritides (p 19). Predictably, occasional cases of rheumatoid arthritis suffer from cutaneous psoriasis, while occasional cases of psoriatic arthritis give positive tests for rheuma-toid factors. These inter-relationships, while conceptually interest-ing, are seldom important practically, provided antimalarial treatment (hydroxychloroquine) is avoided in patients with psoriasis (*see below*).

Treatment

Management closely follows that for rheumatoid arthritis (p 11), apart from avoiding hydroxychloroquine, as this may exacerbate the skin condition. In the more severe cases gold is worth trying, but corticosteroids are even less desirable than in rheumatoid arthritis (their administration complicates management of the skin). When features of spondylitis are present, the principles of treating that condition (p 25), particularly maintenance of regular physical exercise, also apply. In the most severe cases there is an impression (but not proof) that azathioprine (2.5 mg/kg/day) helps the joint condition. It is unclear at present whether or not treatment of the skin condition by methotrexate or 'PUVA' also helps the joints.

Reiter's disease

This is a multisystem disorder, of which an important component is a 'seronegative spondarthritis' (p 19). Typically *'non-specific' urethritis* appears to act as a trigger; less often *bacterial dysentery* is the initial event. A wide variety of extra-articular features may occur, particularly ocular and mucocutaneous. Once 'triggered' the condition tends to recur as self-limiting episodes which can lead to permanent joint deformities.

Aetiology

The course of Reiter's disease suggests that either non-specific urethritis or bacillary dysentery can act as a trigger to set off a multisystem disease (presumably immune-mediated) which is then self-perpetuating independent of the original stimulus. A strong association with HLA-B27 points to genetic susceptibility being important.

Together with conditions such as rheumatic fever (p 97) and Yersinia arthritis (p 91), Reiter's disease has been regarded as an example of 'reactive arthritis' (hence the term 'SARA'—*sexually acquired reactive arthritis*). This concept of a localised infection setting off a widespread, non-infective, polyarthritis harks back to the old notion of 'focal sepsis'. At present it remains only a concept, not a diagnosis, and the exact pathogenetic mechanism remains a matter for speculation. The aetiology and inter-relationships of the seronegative spondarthropathies are discussed further on p 20.

Incidence

Reiter's disease is recognised almost exclusively in males ($M:F = 20:1$). In British hospitals it is probably diagnosed somewhat more often than psoriatic arthritis. It affects mainly young adults, but is seen also in teenage boys. Amongst males who contract 'non-specific' urethritis, those having HLA-B27 are 40 times more likely to develop Reiter's disease.

Clinical features

In the sexually acquired form of the disease the patient usually presents with a mild *urethritis* within two weeks of sexual intercourse (often promiscuous). This may be so mild as to pass unnoticed, or may be associated with a distressing abacterial *haemorrhagic cystitis*. Not infrequently coincidentally acquired gonorrhoea confuses the situation. *Chlamydia trachomatis* can be isolated from 50 per cent of patients with 'non-specific' urethritis, but is not particularly related to the development of Reiter's disease. Further, successful treatment of the urethritis by oxytetracycline does not influence the subsequent course of Reiter's disease. Even though the symptoms of non-specific urethritis may be overlooked by the patient, a thorough genitourinary investigation will usually reveal evidence of anterior and posterior urethritis with associated *prostatitis*. The first urine passed in the morning often contains threads of purulent material.

The *dysenteric type* of Reiter's disease appears to be similar to the sexually acquired form, except that it follows a bowel infection due to *Shigella flexneri, S dysenteriae, S sonnei*, or sometimes other types of diarrhoea.

The 'classical triad' of Reiter's disease refers to the association of three features: urethritis, conjunctivitis and arthritis. Until recently this concept inhibited a better understanding of the condition by suggesting that Reiter's disease was a clear-cut entity. In fact, as explained on page 19, it merges into the other types of seronegative spondarthritis without clear demarcation. Hence the introduction of the term 'SARA' (p 20) to define one clinical group more precisely. For the time being the term Reiter's disease is likely to remain in use. However defined, it may occur in association with a wide variety of associated features.

Arthritis tends to be oligoarticular (one or a few joints), asymmetrical, sometimes very acute in onset, and affects mainly the lower limbs. Sacroilitis and spondylitis may develop at any stage. The initial attack of polyarthritis usually settles within a few months, but many patients experience recurrent attacks. (To what extent these are triggered by further genitourinary or gut infections is unknown.) With repeated attacks, chronic joint deformities develop, particularly pes planus, subluxed metatarsophalangeal joints, clawed toes, sacroilitis and spondylitis (of all degrees, up to complete ankylosis). These more severe cases generally have HLA-B27. Radiologically the joint changes resemble ankylosing spondylitis (p 23) including the tendency for overgrowth of fluffy new bone.

Tenosynovitis is common, involving particularly the Achilles' tendon (p 106).

Conjunctivitis occurs in about one-third of patients. It is generally mild, bilateral and of short duration.

Keratoderma blenorrhagica is a highly characterised skin lesion. It begins as a 2- to 3-mm brown macule which evolves into a papule then a pustule. The soles are the most common site and here the lesion may finish as a circular flap of overhanging dead skin ('iris'). Other sites may be involved, including the scalp and nails (subungual pustulation). Occasionally the lesions become widespread, resembling exfoliative dermatitis, or may evolve into typical psoriasis. On the glans penis in the circumcised similar crusted lesions may appear, while in the uncircumcised moist superficial ulceration (*circinate balanitis*) is the typical lesion.

Mucosal lesions consist of transient painless ulceration of the buccal or pharyngeal mucosa.

Iritis and *cardiovascular lesions* may occur as in ankylosing spondylitis (p 21).

Nervous system involvement is rare, but peripheral neuritis, optic neuritis, neuromyopathy and meningoencephalitis have all been recorded.

Investigations

The ESR reflects the inflammatory activity of the disease. Tests for rheumatoid factor are negative. A majority of patients possess

HLA-B27, particularly those with spondylitis and those with more severe, multisystem disease. Synovial biopsy specimens show a rheumatoid type of reaction (p 4), but polymorphonuclear leucocytes are said to be more numerous.

Management

Non-specific urogenital infection requires treatment in its own right (e.g. oxytetracycline 250 mg six-hourly for 14 days). This is not thought to influence the Reiter's disease. Sexual partners should be investigated. Although the extent to which recurrences are triggered by re-infection is not known, the risks of promiscuous sexual activity should be explained to the patient.

The management of the rheumatic component does not differ from that of any comparable peripheral arthritis or spondylitis. Severe systemic involvement (e.g. neurological) may occasionally justify the use of corticosteroids.

Enteropathic arthritis (colitic arthritis)

Inflammatory bowel disease (ulcerative colitis or Crohn's disease) may be associated with two patterns of arthritis. The one is ankylosing spondylitis (p 20) in which the two conditions appear to progress independently. The other is enteropathic ('colitic') arthritis, which behaves like a complication of the bowel disease. It is the least common form of seronegative spondarthritis (p 19) and usually takes the form of a mild synovitis affecting a few joints in the lower limbs. It never precedes the bowel disease, with which it tends to wax and wane in parallel, and it often improves after successful bowel surgery. The arthritis generally settles spontaneously over a period of weeks or months, and seldom produces permanent joint damage. the pattern of arthritis is not unlike that which occurs with erythema nodosum (p 110), a condition which itself complicates inflammatory bowel disease and may be present at the same time as the arthritis. Unless spondylitis is also present, there is not a clear genetic link with HLA-B27.

5 Systemic connective tissue diseases (collagen-vascular diseases)

For the purpose of differential diagnosis it is convenient to group together as *systemic connective tissue diseases* conditions such as:

Systemic lupus erythematosus (SLE) ✓
Rheumatoid arthritis ✓
Systemic sclerosis (scleroderma) — ✓thickening of dermis/bv's
Polyarteritis nodosa ✓
Other types of arteritis
Polymyositis ✓
Dermatomyositis
Sjögren's syndrome

These enter into the differential diagnosis in any patient presenting with an inflammatory multisystem disease. The group thus requires some convenient collective descriptive term. At one time 'collagen diseases' served this purpose, but the pathological concept underlying that term has been superseded, and most now favour *systemic connective tissue diseases* (an acceptable alternative is *collagen-vascular diseases*).

This grouping is not just one of clinical convenience. There is good evidence that these disorders have pathogenetic and perhaps aetiological factors in common. The obviously shared features include:

Unknown aetiology
Multisystem involvement
Arthritis and vasculitis
Circulating autoantibodies
Evidence of immune complex deposition
Clinical overlap within the group

A common theme is one of *autoimmunity*, and in most of these diseases there is evidence of altered immunological regulation. Much current research aims to test the hypothesis that the altered immune status is a defect in regulation by suppressor T-cells. Even if this is established, the question will remain whether this is a primary immunological fault or whether it is secondary to a viral infection. The association of some cases of polyarteritis nodosa and hepatitis B virus (p 43) and the evidence of animal models of SLE (p 34) point to the interplay of a chronic viral infection plus host susceptibility. But this remains to be established.

The phenomenon of *clinical overlap* (intermediate or mixed clinical pictures, and cases evolving from one clinical category to another) suggest that all these disorders may be variations on a single theme. If this is so, what factors introduce the variation is unknown. This aspect is discussed further on page 59.

In the following chapters these various disorders (except rheumatoid arthritis, already described on p 3) are discussed as separate diseases. This separation is necessary for the clinician because the management and prognosis differ between the various disorders.

Systemic lupus erythematosus (SLE)

SLE is a relatively common disorder affecting particularly young adult females. The pathogenesis probably depends on the deposition of immune complexes containing autoantibodies to nuclear antigens. Almost any tissue may be affected, resulting in widely differing clinical patterns. It exhibits 'overlap' with the other systemic connective tissue diseases (p 32).

Aetiology and pathogenesis

In common with other *systemic connective tissue diseases* the aetiology of SLE is unknown. The best studied lesions are those in the kidney. Here there is strong evidence that immune complexes are filtered out of the circulation to become deposited in the basement membrane, there to fix complement and set off inflammatory changes. It appears likely that such immune-complex depositions may account also for the lesions in other sites such as the skin and joints and it may well represent the common pathological event in this disease.

At least a major component of these immune complexes consists of autoantibodies directed against nuclear material with the corresponding antigen (i.e. DNA + anti-DNA). The conundrum of SLE is whether these autoantibodies represent a response to a viral infection or whether they result from a primary immunological aberration (such as defective T-cell function). Very similar diseases in dogs and in New Zealand mice appear to result from a chronic viral infection in genetically susceptible animals. Other clues to the aetiology may lie in the female preponderance, the precipitating effect of sunlight and certain drugs, and the predisposition to SLE of subjects with defective complement systems.

Pathology

Pathological changes may occur in almost any organ or tissue. They represent varying combinations of four basic changes:

Fibrinoid change consists of eosinophilic strands somewhat resembling fibrin. It may result from different processes, including deposition of plasma proteins.

Collagen sclerosis is seen most obviously in the 'onion skin' concentric fibrosis of splenic arterioles.

Haematoxylin bodies consist of DNA released from cell nuclei (similar to the material in the LE cells—p 133).

Vascular changes affecting arterioles and capillaries are widespread and probably underlie most of the disease manifestations. Fluorescent staining techniques show the presence of immune complexes which are presumed to cause the vasculitis.

Clinical features

In British hospitals one case of SLE is seen for about 20 cases of rheumatoid arthritis. Females outnumber males by 10:1, and the onset is usually during the childbearing years. Familial clustering occurs, but is uncommon. (There is some association with HLA-B8 and DRw3.)

SLE is an episodic disease. Acute, sometimes life-threatening episodes may punctuate prolonged spontaneous remissions. Almost any organ or tissue may be affected.

Joint involvement occurs in over 90 per cent of cases. This ranges from flitting arthralgia to true synovitis similar to rheumatoid arthritis. However, the progressive erosive changes seen in the latter are rare in SLE. *Aseptic necrosis* (p 109) occurs occasionally.

Skin lesions are also extremely common. Most characteristic is the 'butterfly' distribution of erythema on the cheeks and across the bridge of the nose, but almost any type of eruption may occur. Sometimes this takes the form of cutaneous vasculitis, or there may be overlap with the skin changes of dermatomyositis (p 50) or scleroderma (p 39). In the fingers a typical combination is erythema and telangiectasia of the skin at the base of the nail, together with pitted scarring of the pulp. *Photosensitivity* is common. Other features include *Raynaud's phenomenon* and *loss of hair*. Subcutaneous nodules occur but are uncommon.

Relationship to chronic discoid lupus

Discoid lupus behaves like a localised chronic, benign variant of the systemic disease. The erythematous 'butterfly' rash may progress to scarring and pigmentation. The histology is similar to SLE. These patients may possess antinuclear antibodies and occasionally exhibit mild systemic features.

Cardiovascular involvement most often produces *pericardial pain*. There may also be *myocarditis* and *endocarditis*. (These 'Libman-Sacks' vegetations are usually haemodynamically insignificant). *Peripheral vasculitis* may produce widespread ischaemic lesions.

Respiratory involvement most often produces pleural pain. *Effusions, pulmonary infiltrations*, and pulmonary functional changes also occur.

Renal disease is an important cause of death. About 50 per cent of patients show some evidence of kidney involvement. At first this is reversible, later irreversible. Proteinuria, haematuria and hypertension may progress to acute or chronic renal failure, or a nephrotic syndrome. Phases of active and progressive renal disease are marked by high serum DNA-binding values (p 133) and low serum complement levels, believed to indicate immune complex deposition and the need for vigorous treatment

Nervous system involvement also carries sinister implications. *Headache, psychosis* and *epilepsy* are thought to result from cerebral vasculitis. There may also be *peripheral neuropathy*, *myelopathy*, *hemiplegia* or *cranial nerve palsies*.

Eye involvement may manifest as *Sjögren's syndrome* (p 56), or as *papilloedema* or *retinal changes*, including the white exudates known as *cytoid bodies*.

Haemopoietic system involvement most often manifests as *leucopenia* and *anaemia*. Occasionally there may be *autoimmune haemolytic anaemia* with positive Coombs' antiglobulin test (for IgG autoantibodies against red cells), or *thrombocytopenic purpura* similar to the idiopathic type. Another cause of bleeding problems is *circulating anticoagulants*.

Other clinical features include *myopathy*, *abdominal pain*, *splenomegaly* and *lymph node enlargement*.

Drug-induced SLE

Certain drugs, particularly hydrallazine, procainamide, methyldopa and chlorpromazine appear to be capable of inducing a syndrome like SLE, which tends to improve on withdrawing the drug. Also, this drug-induced syndrome tends to be milder, does not lead to renal disease, and is associated with negative DNA-binding tests (p 133).

Less certainly, a wide variety of drugs, including anticonvulsants, antituberculous drugs and antibiotics have been linked with lupus-like syndromes, or at least the appearance of antinuclear antibodies. The interpretation of this is unclear. Conceivably, a straightforward sensitivity reaction to any drug may (like sunlight exposure) trigger a lupus-like attack in a susceptible subject. Whatever the explanation, any drug therapy in lupus patients requires careful consideration.

Relationship to 'lupoid hepatitis'

Liver damage is an uncommon feature of SLE, but young women with *active chronic hepatitis* may develop a syndrome which both clinically and serologically resembles SLE, except that DNA-binding tests are negative. It is probably best regarded as a separate disease rather than a lupus variant.

Investigations

The diagnosis of SLE requires identification of circulating autoantibodies directed against nuclear antigens. Three types of test are employed.

LE-cell test (p 132). This is the original test which defined the disease and provided the first clue to its pathogenesis. Peripheral blood leucocytes are incubated, then smeared and stained. The LE cell is a neutrophil distended with a mass of phagocytosed nuclear material. The mechanism involves antinucleoprotein antibody gaining access into damaged cells, combining with the nuclear surface, fixing complement, and thus attracting polymorphs which strip away the cytoplasm and phagocytose the nucleus. The test is positive in 80 per cent of patients with SLE, particularly in those with severe, active disease. However, it may also be positive in rheumatoid arthritis, other systemic connective tissue diseases, drug reactions and chronic active hepatitis. It is a time-consuming test to perform.

Fluorescent antinuclear antibody (ANA). This rapid and simple test (p 133) is highly sensitive (almost all patients with active SLE give positive results), but positive results may occur in other conditions (*see* LE-cell test above). It is thus a valuable screening test for SLE.

DNA-binding and Crithidia luciliae tests (p 133). Tests for antibodies to native (double stranded) DNA are the most specific serological markers for SLE. They are negative in conditions such as chronic active hepatitis in which the LE-cell and ANA test are positive. This test is relatively insensitive, and a proportion of patients (particularly those with mild or inactive disease) give negative results.

Other autoantibodies. The serum of lupus patients may contain a wide variety of autoantibodies directed against nuclear and cytoplasmic cell components, as well as against lymphocytes, neuronal tissue, clotting factors, etc., and rheumatoid factors.

Serum complement levels may be reduced during periods of active disease, indicating complement consumption during immune complex formation.

Other laboratory tests. The ESR reflects disease activity. Immunoglobulins are generally markedly elevated. The leucopenia and other blood changes have been mentioned above.

Skin biopsy (Band test) of clinically normal, exposed skin examined by fluorescent techniques may show immunoglobulin and complement deposition at the dermoepidermal junction—a useful pointer to the diagnosis.

Diagnosis

The florid case is unmistakable. Difficulty arises when the patient first presents with involvement of a single system. In these circumstances it is a marked elevation of the ESR (or possibly leucopenia or hypergammaglobulinaemia) that is likely to alert the clinician to the need to request an antinuclear antibody screening test. If this is positive, a DNA-binding test may confirm the diagnosis. A skin biopsy (*see above*) may provide useful confirmation.

Difficulty may arise in differentiating SLE from early rheumatoid arthritis in patients with positive antinuclear tests. Features favouring rheumatoid arthritis include radiological joint erosions, subcutaneous nodules, pregnancy remissions, characteristic synovial histology and a negative DNA-binding test. Overlap between SLE and other systemic connective tissue diseases is discussed on page 33.

Treatment

Corticosteroids are the sheet anchor of management, being the only drugs which predictably will suppress SLE inflammation. However, the hazards of prolonged steroid therapy mean that this treatment must be reserved for serious episodes, particularly those involving the brain, kidneys, blood or heart. Such episodes require relatively large doses of prednisolone (40 to 100 mg or more daily). As disease activity subsides the dose is reduced. The objective is either to withdraw prednisolone altogether, or to reduce the maintenance dose to 10 mg daily or less. Long-term dosage above this level places the patient on a collision course for steroid toxicity. For acute life-threatening episodes methylprednisolone can be given as daily intravenous infusions of 1 gm ('*pulse therapy*'). Symptomatic treatment is given concurrently with corticosteroids, and involves use of the same drugs employed for this purpose in rheumatoid arthritis (p 12). Hypertension, epilepsy, renal failure etc., require treatment in their own right.

Despite the use of corticosteroids in a 'fire extinguisher' role to damp down acute episodes, some patients continue to show evidence of continuing disease activity. In these circumstances the patient may be improved by the introduction of an *antimalarial drug* (e.g. hydroxychloroquine 200 mg daily—needing ophthalmological supervision) or the addition of an *immunosuppressive agent* such as azathioprine (2.5 mg/kg).

Predictably, attempts have been made to alter the immunological status of these patients by all available means. However, there is at present no clear indication for plasma exchange (plasmapheresis), removal of white cells by leucopheresis or by thoracic duct drainage, nor the use of antilymphocyte globulin (ALG) or levamisole.

Unnecessary exposure to sunlight and drugs should be avoided.

Pregnancy is not contraindicated unless serious renal disease is present.

Prognosis

About 10 per cent of patients die within five years of diagnosis, many of them having shown early evidence of progressive renal disease. The remainder vary from those who experience little inconvenience from occasional mild manifestations, to others who can manage only on maintenance doses of corticosteroids which make them markedly Cushingoid.

Systemic sclerosis (scleroderma)

In this systemic connective tissue disease the most characteristic clinical feature is hard, waxy thickening of skin, particularly in the hands and face. Internal organs are also affected by collagen sclerosis and vasculitis, leading eventually to renal, pulmonary or cardiac failure. No effective treatment is available.

Aetiology and pathogenesis

The aetiology is unknown, but clinical and serological overlap with other systemic connective tissue disorders (p 32) suggests that systemic sclerosis must in some way be related to other members of this group. Genetic factors appear to be unimportant.

Common to all the structures involved in systemic sclerosis is a process of fibrosis, homogenisation of collagen, sclerosis of blood vessels, and secondary atrophy. During active phases there may be evidence of mild inflammation, with round cell infiltration and oedema, but this later gives way to fibrosis, ischaemia and atrophy. Arteriolar ischaemia appears to be a central event in this process.

Clinical features

The disease usually presents between the ages of 30 and 50 years, and women are affected three times as often as men. The typical history is for a young to middle-aged woman to develop Raynaud's phenomenon, followed later by hardening of the skin of the fingers and mild synovitis of finger joints. At this stage or later, appropriate investigations will reveal evidence of involvement of the oesophagus and other internal organs. Exceptionally, organ involvement may occur in isolation.

Raynaud's phenomenon is an almost invariable accompaniment of systemic sclerosis, preceding the other features sometimes by months or even years. The cyclical colour changes and numbness of the fingers are usually triggered by cold exposure. Although the link with Raynaud's phenomenon is most close with systemic sclerosis, it may occur as a presenting feature of any of the systemic connective tissue diseases (p 32). It is this which lends such sinister significance to the appearance of Raynaud's phenomenon for the first time in adult life.

Skin changes vary from mild thickening and induration of the skin of the finger tips (*acrosclerosis, sclerodactyly*) to extensive involvement of arms, face and upper trunk. The basic change is a hardening and thickening of the skin, giving it a taut, waxy and hidebound texture. This may be accompanied by loss of skin appendages, oedema, altered pigmentation, and atrophy of the digital pulp, giving a hard, tapered finger tip (*poikiloderma*). X-rays may show bone resorption. Facial involvement may produce *microstomia* and fissures radiating from the mouth.

The skin lesions do not have a clear line of demarcation from normal skin. This distinguishes them from *morphoea* and *linear scleroderma* (both of which affect the skin in a somewhat similar manner, but do not involve internal organs).

A rare condition which has to be differentiated from systemic sclerosis is *eosinophilic fasciitis*. In this, widespread skin thickening follows unaccustomed muscular exercise. There is hypergammaglobulinaemia, eosinophilia, and biopsy shows thickening, not of the skin, but of the fascia. It responds to corticosteroids.

Calcinosis may accompany the skin changes, appearing as subcutaneous nodules in the hands and elsewhere, and clearly shows on X-ray.

Telangiectasia also commonly accompanies the skin changes. Occasionally widespread telangiectasia resembling the hereditary haemorrhagic telangiectasia of Osler (but lacking a positive family history) may occur with scleroderma and calcinosis. This association has been called the *Thibierge-Weissenbach* syndrome. The *CRST or CREST* syndrome refers to the association of calcinosis, Raynaud's phenomenon, oesophageal involvement, sclerodactyly and telangiectasia—— thought by some to carry a somewhat better prognosis.

Arthritis of the small joints of the fingers is a common early feature. Mild synovitis of the interphalangeal joints may combine with oedema of the skin and *flexor tenosynovitis* to produce a sausage-shaped digit. Joint changes are not erosive, and normally not progressive or destructive.

Tenosynovitis may be recognised by a leathery crepitus in the flexor tendon sheaths above the wrist during finger movements.

Gastrointestinal tract. The most common internal organ involvement is loss of oesophageal motility. Like Raynaud's phenomenon this occurs early, often without producing symptoms. It may be detected also in patients with other systemic connective tissue diseases. Diagnosis is by contrast radiography. A mouthful of barium swallowed by the patient tilted into a head-down position remains immobile in the aperistaltic oesophagus. When the patient is tilted upright the barium descends into the stomach. Marked involvement may produce reflux oesophagitis and dysphagia.

Less commonly, involvement of other levels of the gut may produce diarrhoea, constipation or malabsorption.

Cardiac involvement is common, but this is usually secondary to pulmonary or systemic hypertension. Occasionally there may be pericarditis, myocarditis or aortic valve lesions.

Lung involvement is also common. Initially this is usually an asymptomatic gas diffusion impairment. Later there may be restrictive lung disease, pleural effusion, or pulmonary hypertension. The incidence of both alveolar and bronchiolar carcinomata may be slightly increased.

Renal lesions are the most important cause of death. There may be very rapid development of malignant hypertension, or the patient may develop chronic renal failure. The propensity of corticosteroids to set off or aggravate hypertension are regarded as an indication to avoid this form of therapy if possible.

Other features include mild polymyositis (p 50), *peripheral neuropathy* and an association with Sjögren's syndrome (p 56). An occasional early symptom is a *5th cranial nerve sensory neuropathy*, with numbness inside the cheek.

Investigations

Elevations of ESR and serum globulins are usually modest, but autoantibodies are commonly found in the serum. A majority of patients have positive fluorescent *antinuclear antibody tests* (p 133), often in a *nucleolar pattern*. Rheumatoid factors may also be detected.

Treatment

No really effective treatment is known. Corticosteroids will suppress the early synovitis, but their use is contraindicated because of the hazard of hypertension. Raynaud's phenomenon is managed by keeping the hands, and body generally, warm. Hypertension must be watched for and treated vigorously if it occurs. Cardiac, renal and respiratory failure, oesophagitis and intestinal malabsorption may all require treatment in their own right.

Course and prognosis

Most patients diagnosed as suffering from systemic sclerosis die from the disease, particularly from renal involvement. The duration of survival from diagnosis varies widely, averaging about five years. Complete remissions have occasionally been reported.

Arteritis: Polyarteritis nodosa

Classification of arteritis

Inflammation involving primarily the arterial wall is termed *arteritis* (or *vasculitis* to include all blood vessels). Various clinical patterns are recognised, ranging from fatal generalised disorders to benign skin conditions. The classification of these is confused, mainly because of ignorance about aetiology and pathogenesis. Arteritis may occur as part of a generalised disorder (e.g. rheumatoid arthritis—p 7) or as a primary pathological event.

The aetiology of these is mainly unknown. In some there is evidence of an immunological disturbance, and deposition of immune complexes in vessel walls may play an important role. The clinical features of these diseases depend on the size and distribution of the vessels involved. They also depend on whether the vasculitis leads to vessel rupture (with haemorrhage) to obstruction (with ischaemia), or to gradual dilatation at the vessel wall (with aneurysm formation).

Polyarteritis nodosa is generally included in the classification of systemic connective tissue diseases (p 32). Other forms of arteritis are less easily classified. For lack of any more logical arrangement, polyarteritis nodosa is described here, while the following two sections deal with four other types of arteritis of particular interest to the rheumatologist. In addition, polymyalgia rheumatica is covered in the same section as giant cell arteritis (p 45) because of the close link between these two conditions. Anaphylactoid (Henoch-Schönlein) purpura is described on page 108.

Polyarteritis nodosa

This serious disease is the best known example of vasculitis, although relatively rare. It affects particularly young and middle-aged males (M:F = 3:1). Medium-sized and small arteries are involved, leading to widespread changes in many organs. Antigen-antibody complex deposition in vessel walls may be the essential pathological event. There is good evidence that in some cases hepatitis B (Australia) antigen is present in the immune complex. In most cases the antigen is unknown.

The lesions are segmental, separated by normal sections, and affect all layers of the arterial wall. There is necrosis, with fibrinoid changes (p 34) and disintegration of the internal elastic lamina. The vessel is surrounded by a cuff of inflammatory cells. Healing is by fibrosis.

Clinical features

A *systemic disturbance* is common, with fever, weight loss and malaise.

Skin lesions range from widespread purpura to patches of skin necrosis. A characteristic appearance of cutaneous vasculitis is *livido reticulosis*—a network pattern of red or purple discolouration in the lower legs. The actual arteritic lesions may be palpable as subcutaneous *nodules*.

Cardiovascular manifestations include *hypertension* (in 50 per cent), *myocardial ischaemia*, *dysrythmias* and *pericarditis*.

Abdominal pain is characteristic. There may also be *bowel infarction* and *mucosal ulceration*. *Liver infarction*, *pancreatitis* and *cholecystitis* can also occur.

Renal involvement is an important cause of death. *Microscopic haematuria* and *hypertension* may progress to acute or chronic renal failure.

Pulmonary lesions include infiltrations or focal necrosis and cavitation. *Asthma* may be a presenting feature, and these patients may have an *eosinophilia* (it has been suggested that such cases represent a relatively benign subgroup of polyarteritis).

Nervous system lesions range from cerebrovascular accidents, such as *hemiplegia* or *visual loss*, to a characteristic form of peripheral neuropathy known as *mononeuritis multiplex*. In this, lesions of vasa nervorum produce ischaemia of individual peripheral nerves. Multiple lesions may add up to a picture which is eventually symmetrical, but the stepwise, assymetrical evolution is highly characteristic. A similar neuropathy may occur as a systemic feature of rheumatoid arthritis (p 7).

Arthralgia or definite synovitis may occur, and there may be features indicating overlap with other systemic connective tissue diseases (p 32).

Investigations and diagnosis

The most characteristic laboratory findings are a *high ESR* and *neutrophil leucocytosis*. Some patients (especially those with pulmonary features) may have an *absolute eosinophilia*. Mild anaemia and hyperglobulinaemia are common, while a minority of patients have positive tests for rheumatoid factors or antinuclear antibodies.

Histology is generally required for diagnosis. This is usually sought by biopsy of a clininically involved tissue, such as skin, kidney, sural nerve or liver.

Arteriography of visceral vessels may show characteristic aneurysms.

Because it involves multiple tissues, polyarteritis often mimics other disorders. The clue to the need to seek histological evidence of arteritis may come from one of the following:

Fever	High ESR
Abdominal pain	Neutrophil leucocytosis
Hypertension	Eosinophilia
Mononeuritis multiplex	Microscopic haematuria

Treatment

Corticosteroids and immunosuppressive drugs are used, but not all cases respond. Active episodes are treated with large doses of prednisolone (60 mg daily or more). If the disease goes into remission the dose is tapered down and, if possible, the drug stopped. If disease activity continues, or if recurrent episodes point to the need for interval treatment, an immunosuppressive drug such as azathioprine (2.5 mg/kg daily) is added. Hypertension may require drug management too.

Prognosis

Mild cases of cutaneous vasculitis can run a benign course. However, polyarteritis with major organ involvement carries a sinister prognosis. Some patients have recurrent episodes over many years, others progress despite treatment and die particularly of renal failure with hypertension.

Giant cell arteritis and polymyalgia rheumatica

Giant cell arteritis has characteristic histological features and tends to involve vessels in the territory of the carotid arteries, particularly scalp vessels.

Polymyalgia rheumatica is a common syndrome occurring in the elderly. It consists of aching myalgic pains in a girdle distribution, severe morning stiffness, general malaise, markedly elevated ESR, and a dramatic response to corticosteroids.

The two conditions frequently coexist and, even in patients with polymyalgia rheumatica who show no clinical evidence of arteritis, biopsy of an apparently normal temporal artery may show the characteristic changes of giant cell arteritis. How to interpret this overlap is unclear. However, whether or not the two conditions are different manifestations of a single disease process, management policy is dictated by the likelihood that they may coexist. The two are here described separately.

Giant cell (temporal or cranial) arteritis

Clinical features

Most patients are over the age of 50, and it is more common in women. *Systemic features*, including fever, malaise and weight loss and muscle aches are common, and there may be the full-blown picture of *polymyalgia rheumatica* (p 47).

Cranial features include *headache*, sometimes severe and intractable. The headache may be generalised or localised to one temporal or occipital area. In the latter case there is sometimes marked local *scalp tenderness*. The temporal arteries may be visibly or palpably thickened with tender areas, sometimes with redness and oedema of the overlying skin. Loss of arterial pulsation is an important sign. Less commonly the occipital artery is involved. Pain may also involve the face, jaw or tongue; sometimes with claudication on chewing.

Ophthalmic arteritis is the very sinister feature of this condition. It may occur at any stage, and lead to irreversible unilateral or bilateral blindness. Ocular pain, diplopia or blurring of vision may give some warning, but blindness can be sudden and complete, due to retinal artery occlusion.

Cerebrovascular arteritis may, less commonly, lead to clinical pictures such as hemiplegia, epilepsy, psychosis, etc.

Investigations

The significant investigation is a *high ESR*, often over 100 mm. However, rarely the ESR may be normal.

Biopsy of an involved segment of scalp vessel establishes the diagnosis. The entire thickness of the artery wall is involved, with necrosis, cellular infiltration, fragmentation of the internal elastic membrane and, characteristically, the presence of multinucleate giant cells. (In patients coming to autopsy similar changes have been observed in branches of the aorta and pulmonary arteries.)

Treatment

As soon as giant cell arteritis is diagnosed (and without waiting for biopsy confirmation) corticosteroids are started immediately to prevent extension of arteritis and the threat of blindness or brain damage. Non-steroidal anti-inflammatory drugs relieve the symptoms but do not prevent blindness.

If there is clinical evidence of active arteritis the starting dose should be at least 100 mg prednisolone daily, and in any case not less than 60 mg. Over the following few weeks the dose is gradually reduced to 10 to 20 mg, provided the patient remains symptom free and the ESR normal. Further gradual reduction should allow eventual withdrawal after several years. Reappearance of clinical arteritis, particularly visual symptoms, is an indication for an immediate return to full doses. Late recurrences may occur after some years.

Polymyalgia rheumatica

Clinical features

Polymyalgia rheumatica occurs mainly in the elderly, and is rare below the age of 50 years. Females are more commonly involved than males (3:1).

The outstanding complaint is *stiffness and aching in a girdle distribution* (neck, shoulders, upper arms, buttocks and thighs). This is associated with prolonged and distressing *morning stiffness*. There is often a marked *systemic disturbance*, including malaise, depression, weakness, weight loss and sometimes low grade fever.

When the shoulder girdle is examined it is found that, although the muscles are somewhat tender, and movements uncomfortable, the shoulder can actually be put through a full range of passive movement. Similarly, neck and hip joint movements are full. Muscle power may be inhibited by discomfort, but true muscle weakness is not a feature. Objective signs of arthritis are normally absent, but the evidence of isotope scanning etc., suggests that there may be an element of synovitis in girdle joints such as the acromioclavicular. Occasionally there may be obvious synovitis of one or more peripheral joints, making differentiation from rheumatoid arthritis difficult.

Any of the features of *giant cell (cranial) arteritis* (p 46) may occur in association with polymyalgia rheumatica, either initially, or appearing during the course of the illness.

The course of polymyalgia rheumatica is unpredictable. Some cases remit within a year or two. Others grumble on for six or more years, or relapse after a period of remission.

Investigations

The only characteristic laboratory finding is *marked elevation of the ESR*, often to over 100 mm. However, rare cases with normal ESR have been observed. There may be a mild anaemia and minor plasma protein changes.

For reasons discussed below, a range of investigations is required to exclude the conditions which may present a 'polymyalgic' clinical picture. This includes *temporal artery biopsy* (p 46).

Aetiology and diagnosis

It is not clear whether polymyalgia rheumatica should be regarded as a separate disease entity. A variety of disorders, including rheumatoid arthritis, polymyositis and myelomatosis, may present a 'polymyalgic' picture initially, although the correct diagnosis becomes apparent with the passage of time. While, amongst those who continue to present features of 'uncomplicated' polymyalgia rheumatica, 25 per cent or more can be shown to have biopsy evidence of giant cell arteritis (p 46). Some cases present with mixed features of both polymyalgia rheumatica and giant cell arteritis; others change from one clinical picture to the other during their illness. Whether one regards polymyalgia rheumatica as a reaction pattern in the elderly which may be triggered by a variety of conditions including giant cell arteritis; or whether one considers all patients with 'uncomplicated' polymyalgia to have associated giant cell arteritis, management strategy is dictated by the possibility that the latter condition is present.

Management

The likelihood of long-term corticosteroid treatment makes it mandatory to establish the diagnosis as firmly as possible at the outset. Many regard this as an indication for performing a temporal artery biopsy initially (under local anaesthetic). A negative biopsy does not exclude giant cell arteritis, but positive histology confirms it.

The symptoms of polymyalgia rheumatica often respond well to non-steroidal anti-inflammatory drugs. However, the likelihood of underlying arteritis, with the threat of blindness, is generally regarded as making corticosteroid treatment obligatory, even when there is no local evidence of arteritis. Also, a dramatic and complete response to starting corticosteroid treatment (e.g. 20 to 30 mg prednisolone daily) provides some confirmation of the diagnosis of polymyalgia rheumatica. (Failure to respond completely is an indication to reconsider the possibility of conditions such as myelomatosis.)

Once remission is achieved the dose of prednisolone is gradually titrated down to the minimum that will maintain freedom from symptoms and a normal ESR. If this requires doses in excess of about 10 mg daily, then the patient is likely to develop problems with steroid side effects. In these circumstances management involves the difficult weighing up of steroid hazards against the small but definite risk of loss of vision. The appearance of visual symptoms (or other local evidence of arteritis) are indications for giving large doses of corticosteroid (e.g. 100 mg prednisolone daily) immediately. Long-term follow-up is required.

Other forms of arteritis

Allergic vasculitis

The separation of allergic vasculitis as a condition different from polyarteritis nodosa (p 43) is somewhat artificial. The pathological and clinical features of the two conditions are basically the same, except that allergic vasculitis tends to be less severe and associated with more florid skin reactions. The differentiation is made by using the term to describe polyarteritis occurring during the course of allergic or hypersensitivity reactions, for example serum sickness or drug reactions.

Treatment is by removing the cause if possible and, if necessary, administering corticosteroids. The prognosis is better than in classical polyarteritis nodosa.

Takayasu's arteritis (Pulseless disease: Aortic arch syndrome)

This rare type of arteritis affects the thoracic aorta and its main branches. It occurs mainly in young women. The histological features are very similar to those of giant cell arteritis.

Clinical features

There is vascular insufficiency in the territory of branches of the thoracic aorta. Claudication in the arms, finger ischaemia, shoulder girdle muscle wasting and a wide variety of ischaemic cerebral syndromes may occur.

Systemic features include malaise and arthralgia. Spondylitis has been reported. Characteristically bruits are heard over the arteries in the neck and arms, and pulsation progressively disappears from these vessels.

Investigations

There is elevation of the ESR, hyperglobulinaemia, and anaemia. *Aortography* establishes the diagnosis by showing occlusion of branches of the thoracic aorta.

Treatment and prognosis

Corticosteroids and surgical vascular reconstruction have been tried, but the prognosis remains poor. Patients die from either myocardial or cerebral infarction.

Wegener's granulomatosis

This rare disease affects young adults and is characterised by a combination of necrotic granulomatous lesions and arteritis affecting particularly the kidneys and respiratory tract.

Clinical features

There are usually marked systemic features with general ill health, arthralgia, fever, anaemia, leucocytosis (often with eosinophilia) and raised ESR.

Necrotic granulomatous lesions in the upper and lower respiratory tract produce sinusitis, rhinitis, pneumonitis, etc. Chest X-rays show multiple opacities which may cavitate.

Focal glomerulonephritis leads to renal failure.

Pathology

The respiratory tract lesions consist of granulomata with areas of necrosis, giant cells, and chronic inflammatory cell infiltration. These are associated with vessels showing necrotising vasculitis. Lesions can be found also in organs outside the respiratory tract. The renal lesion includes necrotising and proliferative glomerulitis.

Treatment and prognosis

A combination of corticosteroids and immunosuppressives may produce prolonged remissions in this disease, which used to be regarded as invariably fatal.

Polymyositis and dermatomyositis

The term *polymyositis* refers to acquired inflammatory disorders of voluntary muscles in which proximal weakness is the cardinal feature.

When this is associated with a particular pattern of skin eruption the term *dermatomyositis* is used.

Classification

A satisfactory classification awaits elucidation of the aetiology and pathogenesis of polymyositis. It seems likely that the term as used at present covers a variety of conditions. The common feature is *diffuse weakness of striated muscles*. The tempo of the disease varies greatly, and many cases show overlap with other systemic connective tissue diseases (p 32). Also, there may be a significant association with malignant disease, and dermatomyositis in childhood is probably somewhat different. For this reason polymyositis is customarily grouped into arbitrary clinical categories such as the following:

1 Pure polymyositis
2 Polymyositis with minor features of other connective tissue disorders
3 Other connective tissue disorders with incidental polymyositis
4 Mixed connective tissue disease
5 Adult dermatomyositis
6 Childhood dermatomyositis
7 Polymyositis or dermatomyositis with malignancy
8 Pure muscle necrosis.

Aetiology and pathogenesis

Affected muscles show fibre degeneration, sometimes with phagocytosis and regeneration. Round cell infiltration may be the most striking feature. Late features include fibrosis and calcification. Children with dermatomyositis, in addition, may show widespread vasculitis with evidence of immune complex deposition.

Experimental evidence suggests that the disease results from an immunological disturbance, with the actual muscle changes being caused by cellular (as opposed to humoral) immune damage. Whether a virus is involved remains a matter of speculation, as does the question of how malignancy might trigger this process.

Clinical features

These conditions are all rare. Women are affected three times more often than men. Apart from childhood dermatomyositis, the midadult years are the most common time of onset. The different types are here described separately, but it must be emphasised that this grouping is arbitrary and there is considerable overlap.

Pure polymyositis

The central feature is voluntary muscle weakness affecting particularly the proximal limb and girdle muscles. Usually there is wasting too, but during the early stages in acute cases there may be an initial phase during which the affected muscles are swollen, doughy and tender, sometimes with oedema of the overlying skin. Later there is atrophy.

In a typical subacute case the patient will usually describe symptoms coming on over a few weeks or months. The distribution of the weakness characteristically causes difficulty in climbing stairs, getting out of a bath, or combing the hair. Spontaneous muscle pain may occur. If the weakness progresses, walking becomes difficult, and the gait waddling. Bulbar muscle involvement is indicated by a nasal voice, dysphagia and choking over food. The most severe cases progress to respiratory paralysis. At any point the process may cease to progress and, after a period which may include exacerbations and remissions, there is some return of muscle power. Healing is partly by fibrosis, leaving the muscles weakened, wasted and indurated. Shortening of muscles may lead, for example, to *flexion deformities* of joints, while a late feature is *subcutaneous calcification*. This can take the form of the finger nodules seen in systemic sclerosis (p 40) or sheets of deep fascial calcification in the buttocks and thighs.

The tempo of this process varies enormously. At one end of the scale it may produce myoglobinuria and death within a few weeks. At the other end of the scale it can be so gradual that the patient does not notice the weakness coming on.

Physical examination reveals proximal limb and girdle muscle weakness, with or without wasting, tenderness, occasionally swelling. Lying flat with the arms folded across the chest (and with counterpressure on the knees by the examiner) the patient cannot rise to a sitting position. Elevation of the abducted arm, or elevated leg, cannot be maintained against resistance. The gait is waddling and the Trendelenberg test (p 128) positive.

The diagnosis requires differentiation from neurological causes of weakness. Points favouring polymyositis are relatively better retention of tendon reflexes, absence of sensory signs, and the symmetrical proximal distribution of weakness.

Although polymyositis is primarily a disease of striated muscle, there may be (smooth muscle) *oesophageal hypomotility* (as in systemic sclerosis—p 41) and *ECG changes or dysrhythmias* indicating cardiac muscle involvement.

The diagnosis of polymyositis is established by three investigations (two of which need to be positive):

Serum enzymes
Electromyography
Muscle biopsy

As these are relevant also to the other clinical groups, they are discussed on page 54.

Polymyositis with features of other connective tissue disorders
The more carefully cases of 'pure' polymyositis are studied, the more often will grounds be found for including them in this group. These features include arthritis, rash, sclerodactyly, Sjögren's syndrome, renal involvement, etc.

Other connective tissue disorders with incidental polymyositis
Electromyographical and serum enzyme studies in patients with rheumatoid arthritis, systemic sclerosis, polyarteritis nodosa and Sjögren's syndrome not infrequently reveal evidence of mild polymyositis which is often clinically inapparent.

Mixed connective tissue disease (MCTD)
This 'overlap' syndrome which includes features of polymyositis SLE and systemic sclerosis—and in which there occurs a characteristic autoantibody—is described on page 59.

Adult dermatomyositis
In dermatomyositis the features of polymyositis occur in association with a characteristic skin eruption. The lesions tend to be erythematous and scaling, and to affect the face, neck, upper arms, knuckles and other extensor prominences. It may be very widespread and associated with cutaneous oedema, sometimes with pruritis. Characteristic features are violaceous ('heliotrope') discolouration of the upper eyelids, with oedema, and atrophic scaling ('collodion patch') lesions over knuckles.

The muscle changes are similar to those in 'pure' polymyositis, but tend to be severe, and systemic features may be prominent. Small joint polyarthritis may be an early feature.

Polymyositis or dermatomyositis with malignancy

Ten to fifteen per cent of patients with polymyositis who are over the age of 40 are found to have an associated malignant neoplasm. This association is slightly more common in males. The most frequent sites are lung, ovary, prostate, breast and gut. Polymyositis or dermatomyositis associated with a malignancy often runs a severe and fatal course.

While patients with polymyositis or dermatomyositis and over the age of 40 should be screened for malignancy, the vigour with which this should be pursued depends on the possibilities for treatment. Whether effective treatment of an associated malignancy improves the underlying polymyositis is uncertain.

Dermatomyositis in childhood

Childhood dermatomyositis is very rare. It differs from the disease in the adult in that—untreated—*muscle contractures and joint deformities* are more common, and *vasculitis* is a prominent feature. The latter may cause abdominal pains and gut haemorrhage or perforation. Vessels in voluntary muscles may show similar changes. If followed up long enough, almost all these children develop *subcutaneous calcification*, sometimes very extensive. There is no association with malignancy.

Muscle necrosis without any inflammatory response

Occasional cases of polymyositis show histological changes consisting of pure muscle necrosis (myolysis) without any evidence of inflammation. Such cases tend to run an acute and unfavourable course, and to be unresponsive to drug therapy. This may well be a different disease from other types of polymyositis.

Investigations

The ESR usually reflects the tempo of the disease, and can be normal in mild cases. The serum may contain a variety of autoantibodies, including rheumatoid factors, antinuclear antibodies, and give a positive LE-cell test.

Muscle enzymes can be detected in the serum in increased quantities after release from damaged muscles. These include:

Creatinine phosphokinase
Aldolase
Lactic dehydrogenase
Transaminases

The first two are more specific for muscle damage and are of value both in the diagnosis of polymyositis and also in following the course of the disease.

Electromyography (EMG) usually allows the diagnosis to be established with certainty. Characteristic features include:

Spontaneous fibrillation
Short-duration polyphasic potentials of low amplitude
Salvos of repetitive potentials

When characteristic these features can differentiate muscle weakness due to polymyositis from that due to lower motor neurone lesions or muscular dystrophy.

Muscle biopsy may reveal some or all of the histological changes mentioned on p 50.

Treatment

Corticosteroids provide the sheet anchor of treatment. For serious cases prednisolone is given in a daily dose of 60 mg or more daily. With improvement (judged by muscle power, serum enzymes and ESR) this is then gradually tapered down. This treatment is likely to have to be continued for months, or years. The second line drugs are *immunosuppressives*, either *azathioprine* (2.5 mg/kg daily by mouth) or *methotrexate* (0.75 mg/kg weekly by intravenous injection). Immunosuppressives are introduced either if there is a failure to respond to corticosteroids or if corticosteroids will control the disease only in a dosage which leads to unacceptable side effects.

Physiotherapy has an important role to play in preventing muscle shortening and deformities. Passive movements and splinting may be required during active phases, followed later by active exercises and functional re-education. These measures are particularly important in children with dermatomyositis. Severely paralysed patients will need intensive total patient care, but this does not present problems peculiar to polymyositis.

Prognosis

Of all patients diagnosed as having polymyositis, about 15 per cent are likely to die as a result of the disease. Amongst the survivors, most will achieve a reasonably normal functional capacity, while a

Sjögren's

minority will be left with varying degrees of more severe disability. The presence of malignancy is predictably ominous. Childhood dermatomyositis is rarely fatal, but can lead to severe deformities, especially if physiotherapy is neglected.

Sicca = dry

Sjögren's syndrome

Sjögren's syndrome is a triad of defective lacrimal secretion (*keratoconjunctivitis sicca*), defective salivary secretion (*xerostomia*), and a *connective tissue disorder*. When the dry eyes and mouth occur in the absence of a systemic connective tissue disorder the term *sicca syndrome* is sometimes applied.

Sjögren's syndrome is encountered mainly in association with other diseases. Whether this represents a 'complication' of the other disease, or whether Sjögren's is a separate condition, perhaps triggered independently by the same aetiological factor, is unknown. Most commonly it occurs in patients with rheumatoid arthritis (30 per cent of whom have evidence of keratoconjunctivitis sicca), but it may occur with any of the systemic connective tissue diseases (p 32) or autoimmune forms of liver or thyroid disease.

Patients with Sjögren's syndrome tend to have a variety of circulating autoantibodies. This is most marked in patients with sicca syndrome alone. These latter patients also tend to have renal and other systemic features, enlargment of lacrimal and salivary glands, and to show lymphatic hyperplasia which may transform into a benign or malignant lymphoma. Immunogenetic studies suggest that such cases may represent a group different from Sjögren's syndrome occurring with rheumatoid arthritis, etc. Tentatively the former cases are referred to as '*primary*', the latter as '*secondary*'. The aetiology of the systemic connective tissue diseases is discussed on page 32.

Pathology

The pathological changes are seen in mucus secretory glands. There is *infiltration with lymphocytes and plasma cells*, followed by *atrophy of acini* and *fibrosis*, with narrowing of ducts. Lymphocytes become aggregated into *follicles with germinal centres*, while duct cells proliferate to form *epi-myoepithelial islands*.

Generalised lymphoid hyperplasia may occur, and there is evidence that what starts as a *polyclonal lymphoid infiltrate* can sometimes progress to a *monoclonal B-cell proliferation* (*see below*).

Clinical features

Females are more commonly affected than men (9:1). Usually the affected salivary and lacrymal glands remain normal in size, but they may become enlarged and firm, although not tender.

Eyes. Superficial gritty irritation and redness are the usual complaints, sometimes with early morning stickiness of the lids. The actual reduction in tear secretion is often not appreciated by the patient. The dryness may lead to *conjunctivitis*, *filamentary keratitis* and *corneal erosions*. Rarely serious visual loss may result from *vascularisation of the cornea*.

Gastrointestinal tract. Dryness of the mouth interferes with forming and lubricating a food bolus. There is difficulty with mastication and swallowing. Items such as dry cream crackers become unmanageable.

The lips and tongue become dry, smooth and sensitive, and dental disease is accelerated.

Gastric and pancreatic secretions are reduced, but seldom to a clinically significant degree.

Respiratory tract. Reduced secretion of mucus predisposes to irritation and infection throughout the upper and lower respiratory tract.

Kidneys. A proportion of patients with Sjögren's syndrome develop *defective renal tubular function*. This usually takes the form of minor impairment of acidification or concentration. Rarely this may progress to the full-blown picture of *renal tubular acidosis* or *nephrogenic diabetes insipidus*.

Genital tract. Vaginal dryness may cause *atrophic vaginitis* and *dyspareunia*.

Lymphomata. In rare instances lymphoid hyperplasia progresses to a point where, on histological grounds, there appears to be a malignant lymphoma; however this is reversed by corticosteroid treatment (*'pseudolymphoma'*). Other cases progress to true malignant lymphomata such as reticulum cell sarcoma.

Other features. A wide variety of other features have been described in association with Sjögren's syndrome, including Raynaud's phenomenon (25%), lymphadenopathy, splenomegaly, peripheral neuropathy, hyperglobulinaemic hyperviscosity syndrome and an increased liability to hypersensitivity reactions to drugs such as penicillin and gold.

Investigations

A variety of blood abnormalities have been described. Apart from raised ESR and anaemia there may be leucopenia, thrombocytopenia and eosinophilia. A wide range of *autoantibodies* may be present, including rheumatoid factors, antinuclear antibodies, as well as antibodies reacting with salivary duct cells, thyroglobulin and mitochondria etc. Hyperglobulinaemia may be very marked.

Biopsy of the buccal mucosa is a minor procedure which provides excellent material for detecting the characteristic changes in mucous glands.

Sialography. Retrograde injection of contrast medium into the parotid gland shows characteristic saccular changes.

Schirmer's test measures tear secretion. A strip of 5-mm wide filter paper is left hooked in the lower conjunctival sac with the eyes lightly closed. After 5 minutes at least 15 mm of the paper should be moist.

Rose Bengal or fluorescein drops instilled into the conjunctival sac will reveal the superficial corneal ulcerations of keratoconjunctivitis sicca.

Slit lamp examination shows strands of mucus and corneal epithelium adhering to the cornea and bulbar conjunctiva (*filamentary keratitis*).

Diagnosis

Once Sjögren's syndrome is suspected the diagnosis is readily established by the Schirmer test, Rose Bengal and slit lamp examinations. Histological confirmation by buccal gland biopsy is seldom necessary.

Salivary and lachrymal gland enlargement with reduced secretions may result from sarcoidosis, leukaemia or lymphomatous infiltration. *Salivary gland biopsy* may be required to establish the diagnosis. The situation is confusing, for Sjögren's syndrome itself may rarely progress to a lymphoma. The terminology is confused too: *Mickulicz's syndrome* is lymphomatous infiltration of the lachrymal and salivary glands producing dryness, while *Mickulicz's disease* was the term previously used to describe Sjögren's syndrome.

Prognosis

In most patients Sjögren's syndrome remains no more than a minor eye and mouth problem.

Rarely the eye dryness may become more troublesome, or even lead to more serious sequelae. Even more rarely, renal or neoplastic complications—or amyloidosis—develop.

Treatment

Treatment is symptomatic. Frequent use of 1 per cent methyl cellulose eye drops ('artificial tears') and glycerine mouth washes can be helpful.

Dry eyes are particularly vulnerable to wind and dust. Spectacle frames with side shields—or goggles—are worth trying in severe cases.

Overlap syndromes: Mixed connective tissue disease

On page 33, in discussing the classification of the systemic connective tissue diseases, attention was drawn to the *overlap* between these various disorders. Some patients present pictures intermediate between two or more conditions, others appear to evolve from one into another during the course of their illness.

Should one therefore regard all these disorders as variations on one basic disease? For the clinician it is certainly necessary to be more precise in diagnosis, for both prognosis and treatment differ between these sub-divisions. Amongst the various patterns of overlap there is one which is currently emerging with a claim for recognition as a separate disorder—that is *mixed connective tissue disease*.

Mixed connective tissue disease (MCTD)

This overlap syndrome includes features of SLE, scleroderma and polymyositis. Renal disease is uncommon, the prognosis favourable, and the response to corticosteroids good. The serum contains high titres of an autoantibody to nuclear ribonucleoprotein.

Clinical features

Young adult females are mainly affected. They usually present with features of SLE: arthritis, rash, serositis, and fever, or with proximal muscle weakness as in polymyositis. Others present with Raynaud's phenomenon, swollen scleroderma-like hands and oesophageal hypomobility. The overlap pattern may be present from the beginning or evolve during the course of the disease.

Joints. Arthralgia is almost invariable. Most develop true synovitis, usually non-erosive, but occasionally rheumatoid-like erosive changes and even nodules occur.

Skin. Raynaud's phenomenon may antedate other complaints. Characteristically the skin of the hands is swollen and taut. There may also be skin changes of scleroderma with telangiectasia, or features more typical of SLE or dermatomyositis.

Muscles. Any severity of polymyositis may occur from subclinical grades detected only on electrical studies (EMG) to gross muscular weakness.

Other features. Any of the clinical features associated with SLE, polymyositis or systemic sclerosis may occur. However, notably rare are the serious renal and neuropsychiatric features of SLE and the progressive visceral changes of systemic sclerosis.

Investigations
In general the results of most laboratory investigations are a predictable mix of those obtained in SLE, polymyositis and systemic sclerosis.

The exception is the autoantibody pattern. Clinical features alone would not establish MCTD as a separate entity. The claim for that rests largely on the presence in the serum of high titres of an antibody directed against nuclear ribonucleoprotein (*see* Appendix C, p 134).

A pointer to the presence of this autoantibody may first come when the fluorescent ANA test shows a speckled pattern in high titre. In itself this indicates the presence of antibodies to *extractable nuclear antigens* (ENA). Antibodies to one of these ('Sm') are characteristically found in SLE, while antibodies to nuclear ribonucleoprotein (sensitive to RNAse and to trypsin) are the marker for MCTD.

Treatment
Corticosteroid treatment appears to be effective and should be tried once the diagnosis is made.

Prognosis
The prognosis seems to be better than would be anticipated in a disorder representing a mix of SLE, systemic sclerosis and polymyositis.

The claim for MCTD to be regarded as a separate entity is still being field tested. If the original observations are confirmed it will remain to decide whether this is a separate disorder with better prognosis, or whether in SLE-like illnesses antibodies to nuclear RNP confer some protection.

6 Osteoarthritis

Like engine bearings, biological joints sometimes fail. This *degenerative joint disease* is referred to as osteoarthritis (or osteoarthrosis) when it affects synovial joints, while the somewhat similar process affecting the intervertebral joints is called spondylosis (pp 68, 69). Minor degrees of these changes are increasingly common with advancing years and almost universal in old age. Despite the term 'degenerative', minor inflammatory features are common.

Aetiology and pathogenesis

The structural arrangement of smooth hyaline cartilage which caps the ends of the bone forming a synovial joint (p 2) provides an almost frictionless bearing with sufficient elastic cushioning to absorb normal mechanical stresses.

It is likely that the critical changes in osteoarthritis take place in the hyaline cartilage. This leads, on the one hand, to roughening of the bearing surface, with increased friction and abrasion. On the other hand, the cushioning (mechanical energy absorption) becomes impaired, so that the underlying bone is damaged. What starts this process is unknown. The ageing chondrocyte may synthesise less matrix (proteoglycan), the collagen fibres may suffer fatigue fractures or, conceivably, the bone itself may lose its elasticity through the healing of trabecular microfractures. The clinical observation that abnormal mechanical stress produces premature osteoarthritis, points to a central role for mechanical trauma in this process. Articular cartilage has only very limited powers of repair. Nevertheless, minor degenerative changes are not necessarily progressive, and are compatible with symptom-free functioning of a joint over many years. If the process does become progressive, then continued use leads to increasing damage. This is clinical osteoarthritis. Progressive damage probably results from a combination of abrasion of the roughened cartilage surfaces and digestion by various autolytic enzymes released from damaged chondrocytes.

The earliest visible change is roughening of the cartilage surface—*fibrillation*. This is followed by progressive thinning of the cartilage until bare bone is exposed. Before this stage is reached, however, reactive bone changes will have been obvious on X-rays. The bone ends become *sclerotic* with irregular outgrowths of bone round the margin—*osteophytes*. In addition, spaces appear within the cortex which are filled with connective tissue—'*cysts*'.

Mechanism of symptoms

As explained on page 2, joint pain probably arises mainly from collagenous structures such as capsule and ligaments. In osteoarthritis the altered anatomy perhaps makes these structures more vulnerable to stresses and stretching. Certainly mechanical strains tend to trigger painful episodes in weight-bearing osteoarthritic joints. But there may be other mechanisms.

Wear particles have to be cleared from the joint by phagocytosis, a process which will lead to release of chemical mediators of inflammation. In addition, microcrystals of hydroxyapatite (the mineral element of bone) have been identified in osteoarthritic joints. It is possible that these cause a low grade 'crystal synovitis' (p 78). Finally, there is some suggestion that in advanced osteoarthritis intramedullary venous pressure may contribute a dull bone ache. These various theories do not explain why such a wide range of operative surgical procedures on (or even beside) osteoarthritic joints often provide immediate, if short-term, pain relief. However, the effectiveness of resurfacing damaged bone ends points to high stresses within bone being important.

Clinical features

Minor degenerative changes are universal after middle age, and may begin during the third decade. Only a minority develop clinical osteoarthritis, nevertheless, this is the most common cause of joint pains. Women are affected more often than men (3:2), and are particularly liable to develop the characteristic 'nodal' pattern in the hands (*see below*). This runs in families as an autosomal dominant. Apart from this, familial clustering is not impressive. The term 'secondary osteoarthritis' is used to describe degenerative changes resulting from abnormal stresses such as altered weight transmission following malalignment of a fracture (or damage from previous inflammatory arthritis).

Osteoarthritis producing complaints most often affects the hands, hips or knees. The first tarsometatarsal joint is also commonly involved (it transmits the weight of the whole body). In fact, any joint may be affected. However, primary osteoarthritis is rare in the wrist—a useful point of differentiation from inflammatory conditions such as rheumatoid arthritis.

Symptoms

Osteoarthritis is a purely local condition and produces no systemic disturbance. Quite marked changes may produce few symptoms; witness the unsightly, gnarled hands of some older women with nodal osteoarthritis. More gross Heberden's nodes (see below) may be uncomfortable, sometimes with acutely inflamed cystic swellings (relieved by aspiration and corticosteroid injection). Osteoarthritis of the thumb carpometacarpal joint may be painful and interfere with grip.

Predictably the more serious problems arise in weight-bearing joints, particularly the hip and knee. At first pains occur during and following activity. Later there is a continuous dull ache which may interfere with sleep. Stiffness is a feature. The joint 'gels' on resting and has to be loosened up by activity. However, the prolonged early morning stiffness of conditions such as rheumatoid arthritis is absent. Minor stresses may lead to worsening of the symptoms for a few days. An important cause of diagnostic error is when hip joint pain is falsely localised to the knee (via the obturator nerve which supplies both joints).

Signs

The characteristic findings in an osteoarthritic joint are *bony swelling* and *crepitus*. Later, movements become restricted in range and painful. Conspicuously absent is the synovial swelling typical of rheumatoid arthritis. However, evidence of mild inflammation can usually be detected as slight warmth of the overlying skin and a synovial effusion. Localised tender 'trigger points' may be identified, possibly indicating sites of soft tissue strains (p 63). With advanced joint destruction there may be *coarse grating crepitus, flexion p formities, instability* and *subluxation*.

The pattern of osteoarthritis in the hand of middle-aged and c women is highly characteristic (Fig 6.1). This *familial nodal oste thritis* affects the terminal interphalangeal joints of the fingers, pea-sized osteophytes (Heberden's nodes) at the base of the di phalanx on either side of the dorsal surface. The affected jc

Osteoarthritis, unlike Rheumatoid
arthritis is rare
in the wrist.

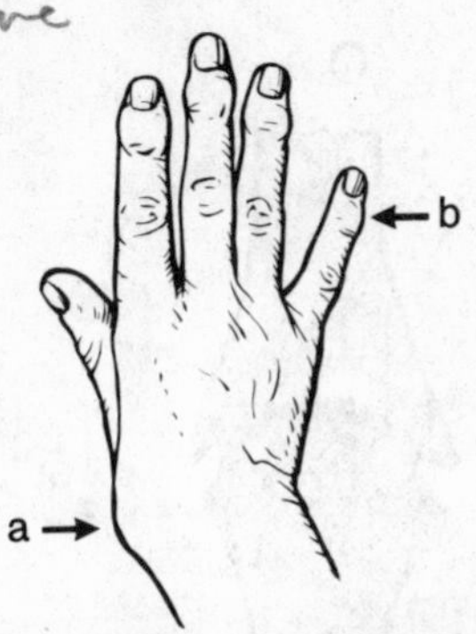

Figure 6.1 Typical appearance of osteoarthritis in the hand of a middle-aged
or elderly woman. Osteophytes of the terminal interphalangeal joints (b) are
known as Heberden's nodes. Osteoarthritis of the first (thumb) carpometacarpal joint (a) gives the appearance of a 'square hand' resulting from (i)
swelling of the joint, (ii) adduction deformity of the first metacarpal bone
and (iii) wasting of nearby small muscles

usually also has a flexion or lateral deformity. Less commonly the
interphalangeal joints are involved (*Bouchard's nodes*). Also characteristic is osteoarthritis of the *thumb carpometacarpal joint*. This can
be painful and disabling. In advanced cases it gives the hand a *square*
appearance (due to bony swelling of the joint, adduction deformity of
the metacarpal and wasting of the surrounding small muscles). The
joint between the trapezium and scapoid may be affected too, but
primary osteoarthritis of the wrist is otherwise uncommon (cf.
rheumatoid arthritis).

Investigations

Osteoarthritis is a local joint disease without systemic features. The
sedimentation rate and haemoglobin are not affected, and tests for
rheumatoid factors and antinuclear antibodies are negative.

Synovial fluid examination is not particularly helpful, except to
exclude the presence of crystals. The cells and protein content have
the characteristics of a non-inflammatory fluid (p 135).

Synovial biopsy also reveals non-specific features. Minor, low-grade
inflammatory changes may be present.

X-rays are useful both in establishing the diagnosis of osteoarthritis
and in grading its severity. The main features have been mentioned

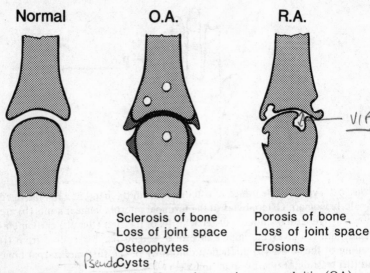

Sclerosis of bone
Loss of joint space
Osteophytes
Pseudo Cysts

Porosis of bone
Loss of joint space
Erosions

Fig 6.2 Comparison of the X-ray changes in osteoarthritis (OA) and rheumatoid arthritis (RA). This diagram does not show the alterations in periarticular bone density: sclerosis in OA, porosis in RA

on page 63. Table 6.1 and Fig 6.2 contrast these with the changes seen in rheumatoid arthritis (p 9).

Loss of radiological 'joint space' (actually radiolucent articular cartilage) is a non-specific feature of joint damage. The other features generally serve to differentiate inflammatory from degenerative arthritis.

Table 6.1 X-ray changes in osteoarthritis contrasted with those in rheumatoid arthritis

	Rheumatoid arthritis	*Osteoarthritis*
Bone density	Porosis	Sclerosis
Joint space	Reduced	Reduced
Erosions	+	0
Cysts	0	+
Osteophytes	0	+

Management

The major advance in the treatment of osteoarthritis has been the development of *prosthetic joint replacements*. At the hip and the knee this operation can provide complete relief of pain and excellent function. However, uncertainties about the life of these devices, and the unavoidable risks of infection and loosening, mean that the procedure is undertaken only when pain and functional problems demand it.

Short of surgery there is still much that can be done for the patient with osteoarthritis. *Drugs* are somewhat less effective than in in-flammatory joint disease, but the same range of analgesics and non-steroidal anti-inflammatory agents used in rheumatoid arthritis (p 12) are used also in osteoarthritis. 'Slow-acting' drugs such as gold and penicillamine are not used, nor are systemic corticosteroids.

Joint aspiration and local corticosteroid injection. Draining a large effusion and injecting (for a knee) 50 to 100 mg of hydrocortisone acetate can provide considerable relief, but this usually lasts only for days, occasionally for weeks. An irritable thumb carpometacarpal joint may also respond well to a local corticosteroid injection.

When pain in an osteoarthritic knee appears to arise from tender soft tissue trigger sites (p 64) relief may be obtained by infiltrating these with local anaesthetic and corticosteroid.

Physiotherapy has an important role in the treatment of osteoarthri-tis. The rationale for its use is that arthritis produces wasting and weakness of muscles acting across the affected joint. Because joint stability depends to a large extent on the pull of these muscles, this wasting leads to joint instability and hence to increased vulnerability to the 'strains' which are believed to produce both pain (p 63) and progressive joint damage. The only proven method of increasing muscle bulk and strength is *active exercises against resistance*. These need not involve actual movement of the joint. Thus the familiar 'quadriceps drill' can be performed within a plaster cast.

More often, exercises involve moving the joint against resistance. Such active exercises, normally undertaken under the supervision of a physiotherapist, can improve function, increase the range of movement and (indirectly) reduce pain.

Electrical methods of warming the tissues (such as radiant heat or short-wave diathermy) can—like a hot water bottle—provide tem-porary pain relief. The popular belief that electrotherapy does more than this is unsubstantiated.

Splints and walking appliances may be needed for patients with severely affected joints.

7 Spondylosis and disc lesions

Degenerative changes affecting peripheral synovial joints are referred to as *osteoarthritis* (p 62). When a somewhat similar process takes place in the spine it is known as *spondylosis*. This chapter deals with spondylosis and the related subject of mechanical lesions of intervertebral discs.

Spondylosis and disc lesions represent a range of closely linked conditions. At one end of the scale, in younger patients, a disc may protrude to give local pain and pressure on a nerve root. At the other end of the scale, in elderly patients, shrinkage of multiple discs and secondary bony overgrowth may also give local pain as well as nerve root irritation. Such lesions are extremely common. The vast majority occur either in the lower cervical or lower lumbar segments of the spine. Thus, if a nerve root is irritated this will give, in the cervical spine, arm pain ('brachial neuralgia') or, in the lumbar spine, leg pain ('sciatica').

Backache with or without leg pain, and neck ache with or without radiation into the arm are both excessively common and also difficult to diagnose precisely. Widely different pathological mechanisms are implied in some of the popular terms: 'fibrositis', 'muscle strain', 'sacroiliac strain', 'postural backache', 'brachial neuritis', etc. In fact, if well defined diseases such as infections, neoplasms, ankylosing spondylitis etc., are excluded, the vast majority of these pains are probably caused by the spectrum of pathological changes defined as disc disease and spondylosis.

Pathological changes (Fig 7.1)

The intervertebral disc consists of a strong fibrous outer rim, the *annulus fibrosus*, enclosing a jelly-like centre, the *nucleus pulposus*. The latter has an affinity for water and swells within the annulus to form an effective shock absorber. With age this water content decreases and the discs shrink. The disc is sandwiched between plates of hyaline cartilage on the vertebrae.

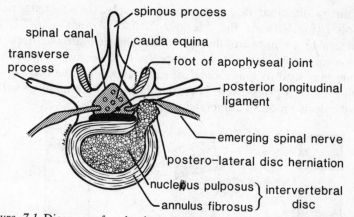

Figure 7.1 Diagram of a lumbar vertebra from above. Note how the situation of the emerging nerve root makes it vulnerable to compression between the disc and the posterior (facetal, apophyseal) joint. Disc geometry favours posterior disc protrusions (herniations). However, the posterior longitudinal ligament tends to direct these posterolaterally (as illustrated here)

Acute disc protrusions may result from indirect trauma, as in lifting. The annulus tears, allowing the nucleus to herniate out. Both in the cervical and lumbar segments disc geometry determines that protrusions tend to be directed posteriorly. However, the strong *posterior longitudinal ligament* usually diverts this posterolaterally, in which direction lies the emerging nerve root in its dural sheath (Fig 7.1). Anterior and lateral protrusions avoid nerve roots, while the rare central posterior protrusions may compress the cord in the cervical region, or cauda equina in the lumbar region (the cord ends at the level of L1) and may even produce CSF block. Small vertical protrusions into the vertebral bodies produce characteristic radiological *Schmorl's nodes*. Whether these produce symptoms is unknown.

Spondylosis refers to all degenerative changes in the spine. The apophyseal (facetal) joints undergo changes similar to synovial joints elsewhere. In the joints between the bodies of the vertebrae, age-related changes in the disc, such as shrinkage, are accompanied by (and perhaps cause) irregular bony outgrowths from the vertebral bodies. Striking spurs, rims and 'beaks' of bone grow out from the edge of the vertebrae. The shape and position of these suggest that their outgrowth may be stimulated by elevation of the periosteum by displaced disc material. Predictably, the emerging nerve roots (lying between the disc and the facetal joint—Fig 7.1) are vulnerable to pressure through these changes. In the neck the *vertebral artery* may also be compressed, while inward growth of bone may lead to *spinal canal stenosis*. The initial diameter of the spinal canal is probably an important factor in determining whether spondylosis produces compression of the contents.

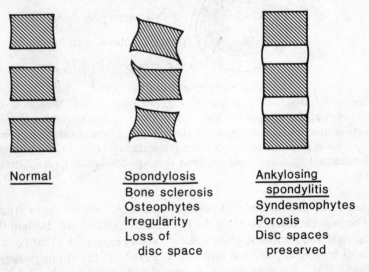

Normal

Spondylosis
Bone sclerosis
Osteophytes
Irregularity
Loss of
    disc space

Ankylosing
    spondylitis
Syndesmophytes
Porosis
Disc spaces
    preserved

Figure 7.2 Comparison of the spinal X-ray changes in spondylosis and ankylosing spondylitis. This diagram does not show the changes in bone density: sclerosis in spondylosis, porosis in ankylosing spondylitis

X-rays most clearly reveal the changes of spondylosis, the spine taking on a gnarled and distorted appearance with reduction in intervertebral disc spaces (Fig 7.2). The osteophytes tend to be horizontal, in contrast to the vertical syndesmophytes of ankylosing spondylitis (p 23).

Ankylosing hyperostosis (Forrestier's disease) is a common, usually symptomless, radiological finding in older patients. Particularly in the dorsal spine, this appears as gross spondylotic bony overgrowth, sometimes with bridging between vertebrae. However, the disc spaces are well preserved. The changes tend to be more marked on the right side of the spine. New bone may be laid down also at other sites.

Clinical features

In both the cervical and lumbar regions there is a spectrum of clinical presentations ranging from acute disc displacement to chronic spondylosis. For clarity the two are described separately. In practice features of both are often combined. At both sites the main complaint is usually local pain with or without pain extending down the arm or leg. The pattern of sensory symptoms and neurological signs resulting from compression of nerve roots is set out in Table 7.1. Disc and/or spondylotic syndromes in the dorsal spine do occur, but are rare, and will not be described separately.

Table 7.1 Functional distribution of cervical and lumbar nerve roots likely to be involved in disc lesions (simplified)

Root	Motor	Sensation	Reflexes
C5	Shoulder abduction	Deltoid region	Biceps
C6	Wrist extension	Thumb and index finger	Supinator
C7	Elbow extension	Middle finger	Triceps
C8	Finger flexion	Little and ring fingers	0
T1	Small hand muscles	Ulnar aspect of forearm	0
L2	Hip flexion and adduction	Front of thigh	0
L3	Knee extension	Front of knee	Knee
L4	Ankle dorsiflexion	Inner shin	(Knee)
L5	Toe dorsiflexion	Outer shin; dorsum of foot	0
S1	Knee flexion; foot plantar flexion	Outer border of foot; sole	Ankle

Cervical disc protrusion

Acute cervical disc protrusions occur mainly in young people. The condition may follow trauma. More often the patient awakes with a stiff, painful neck, the head being held to one side (*acute torticollis*). Examination reveals marked asymmetrical spasm of the neck muscles, usually with no evidence of nerve root or spinal cord compression. Occasionally there may be symptoms and signs of a C7 root lesion (less often C6 or C8—*see* Table 7.1). The condition almost invariably settles spontaneously, but rarely it may persist for up to three months. Treatment is by rest and analgesics. A *plastazote collar* or *traction* (10 to 15 kg) may be helpful. Spinal cord compression is rare. If there are suspicious features (sphincter disturbance, extension plantar response, etc.) myelography using a radio-opaque contrast medium is indicated. As with all the conditions discussed in this chapter, myelography is undertaken when (a) surgical intervention is contemplated or (b) when it is felt necessary to exclude alternative pathological lesions, such as neoplasms or infection.

Cervical spondylosis

This extremely common condition affects particularly the middle-aged. Neck pains, with or without radiation down one or both arms, tend to be aggravated by neck movements. There may be acute episodes resembling disc protrusions, but more often the picture is one of chronic grumbling aches which wax and wane over weeks or months. A small minority develop evidence of long tract involvement due to cord compression, or interference with vertebral artery flow leading to vertigo on looking upwards, or 'drop attacks' precipitated by neck movements.

Examination reveals painful limitation of neck movements (which may provoke pain radiating into an arm). In a minority there is a neurological deficit, most commonly in the distribution of C5, 6 or 7 (Table 7.1). Occasionally there is evidence of cord compression in the form of extensor plantar responses or other long tract signs.

In this age group X-rays are likely to show evidence of cervical spondylosis (p 70), particularly at the level of C5, 6, 7, but the correlation between these and symptoms is often poor. Oblique views sometimes show osteophyte encroachment on a nerve root foramen, and it may be possible to form a rough estimate of the spinal canal diameter.

The diagnosis of cervical spondylosis has often to be made on rather imprecise grounds. The clinical picture can be mimicked by infective or neoplastic lesions, and careful history taking, general examination and investigations such as a blood count or ESR may provide important clues. Radiological changes do not provide positive evidence that neck pains are due to spondylosis. However, X-rays are an important means of seeking other lesions. The CSF may show a modest elevation in protein content.

The prognosis is unpredictable. A very small proportion of these patients develop cord compression, or serious nerve root lesions. The majority experience episodes of neck and/or arm pain which lasts for days or weeks. Generally the condition is not progressive, and prolonged or permanent remissions are not uncommon.

Treatment. A very small proportion of cases require surgical relief of cord compression or osteophytic encroachment on a nerve root.

Short of surgery there is no predictably effective method of relieving pain, apart from analgesics and local heat. However, individual patients may obtain relief from one or other of the traditional remedies: rest, wearing a plastazote collar, using a 'butterfly' pillow at night, traction or manipulation. These are usually tested in turn, and sometimes none is helpful. Before prescribing traction or manipulation it is mandatory to X-ray the neck and exclude an infective, neoplastic or rheumatoid lesion. In the presence of any neurological deficit these methods of treatment are potentially dangerous.

Acute lumbar disc protrusion

Typically there is a history of 'straining' the back, as in lifting, accompanied by immediate lumbar pain, which may 'lock' the patient by muscle spasm. Either immediately or hours or days later the pain may spread to the buttock, then down the back of one leg as 'sciatica'. Occasionally sciatica occurs in the absence of backache. Characteristically the pain is aggravated by flexing the lumbar spine, by turning over in bed, or by manoeuvres which increase intraspinal pressure, such as sneezing or straining at stool. There may, in addition, be symptoms of nerve root involvement, such as altered sensation or muscle weakness. Bilateral neurological symptoms, multiple segment involvement, and, particularly, sphincter disturbances suggest cauda equina lesions and demand urgent investigation.

Examination is likely to show scoliosis (due to muscle spasm), tenderness of the lumbar spine, and painful restriction of lumbar spine flexion, but with lateral bending better retained. Neurological examination may reveal evidence of a nerve root lesion (Table 7.1). Most often involved is the S1 root due to L5/S1 disc lesions. Above this level lesions are progressively less common.

A characteristic sign is painful limitation of *straight leg raising* (Lesègue's sign). With the patient lying flat on his back, hip joint flexion is first tested with the knee on that side flexed (to avoid stretching the sciatic nerve). Next the straightened leg is raised passively (and gently!) from the bed by the examiner grasping the foot. Normally the hip can be flexed painlessly in this way to 90°. With a lower lumbar disc protrusion pressing on a nerve root straight leg raising is limited by a nerve root type of pain. Dorsiflexion of the foot when the leg is partly raised has an additive effect by further stretching the sciatic nerve. Straight leg raising is recorded as degrees of hip flexion. It provides a reproducible means of following the progress of sciatica.

The comparable '*femoral stretch test*' may be positive with higher lumbar disc lesions. With the patient lying prone the knee is flexed to 90°. Extension of the hip joint produces an additive effect in stretching the femoral nerve.

What has been said about investigation of cervical disc lesions (p 71) applies also to lumbar lesions. Standard X-rays are of value mainly in excluding other lesions. The ESR, blood count etc. also serve to exclude the various infective, neoplastic, metabolic and other lesions which may mimic a disc protrusion. If a focal bone lesion is suspected, a radioisotope bone scan is worth performing, while HLA-B27 testing (p 24) may occasionally be indicated. Myelography using a radio-opaque contrast dye is undertaken only if surgery is contemplated or if some other lesion is suspected. Neoplasms such as neurofibromata or meningiomata are likely to produce very high CSF protein values. Modest elevation may result from uncomplicated disc lesions.

Untreated, individual attacks last days, weeks or months, then subside. One episode predisposes to further attacks. Recurrent episodes may merge into the picture of lumbar spondylosis (p 75).

Treatment. As the natural history of individual attacks is for spontaneous improvement (the protrusion presumably 'heals'; it does not return into the disc space) the first line of treatment is bed rest and analgesic/anti-inflammatory drugs. Local heat may also be helpful. Traditionally a flat (boarded) bed is prescribed, but it would seem more logical to allow whatever mattress the patient finds most comfortable. As the pain settles (in days or weeks) the patient is progressively mobilised. A lumbar (Goldthwaite) corset is found helpful by some, presumably because it inhibits flexion. Sometimes a plaster of Paris cast is employed to provide ambulant lumbar immobility, but many patients find this very difficult to manage. Physiotherapists teach a routine of 'back life' to patients who have experienced lumbar disc lesions. The objective is to avoid manoeuvres liable to provoke recurrences, and to use legs and back correctly in lifting.

The vast majority of cases settle spontaneously, over days or weeks. However, if severe sciatic pain persists, particularly in the presence of a neurological deficit, or if there is suspicion that some other pathology may be present, or if there is evidence of cauda equina compression (sphincter disturbance, multiple roots involved, or peri-anal sensory changes etc.), then myelography using a radio-opaque contrast dye is indicated. If this shows a filling defect at the appropriate level, then operative *discectomy* will predictably relieve the leg pain. However, neurological deficits may persist, and the operation does not necessarily relieve backache. Thus the main indication for myelography (apart from suspicion of a tumour) is *persisting severe leg pain*. The late results of surgery performed for less than adequate indications point to the need to persist with conservative management. This may involve six weeks complete bed rest.

Other forms of treatment remain controversial. *Epidural analgesia* (infiltration of the extradural space with dilute local anaesthetic— with or without corticosteroid—via either the lumbar route or sacral hiatus) provides immediate relief of sciatica pain for at least some hours. With various modifications this has enjoyed popularity both as a method of assessment and as treatment. *Lumbar traction* applied in a variety of ways is extensively used in some units, while many physiotherapists favour *exercises designed to strengthen back muscles*. Finally, *manipulation* is discussed below (p 76) in connection with lumbar spondylosis. The widely differing policies of management advocated point, firstly, to the fact that no one form of treatment is reliably and predictably effective and, secondly, to the fact that there is a great need for controlled clinical trials.

Lumbar spondylosis and low back pain

Radiological spondylotic changes are present in the lumbar spine of everyone from middle age onwards. However, the correlation between these and backache is poor, so it remains uncertain to what extent the excessively common complaint of low back pain should be ascribed to lumbar spondylosis. Other mechanisms have been proposed: fibrositis, muscle strain, postural backache, fat herniation, sacroiliac strain, etc. For these there is even less convincing evidence. It therefore appears likely that most low backache—once infective, neoplastic and metabolic lesions, congenital/anatomical defects and HLA-B27-related conditions (p 19) are excluded—is due to lumbar spondylosis and associated disc lesions.

If this view is accepted, then the symptoms of lumbar spondylosis range from chronic low back pain which waxes and wanes, to more acute episodic backache which may be provoked by lifting or other strains. In addition there may be root pains of the type described above under disc lesions. These pains tend to be aggravated by bending, sneezing, rolling over in bed, and by activity generally. A small proportion of patients develop cauda equina involvement.

On examination there is likely to be painful limitation of lumbar spine flexion (with lateral bending better retained—cf. ankylosing spondylitis) and some restriction of 'straight leg raising' (p 73). The lumbar spine is often tender. With nerve root pressure there may be a neurological deficit (Table 7.1).

Investigations are obligatory to exclude the more serious conditions which may mimic 'mechanical' backache, but there is no positive means of establishing that spondylosis is the cause of backache. Careful history taking, physical examination and investigations are all important in excluding conditions such as secondary carcinoma (breast, prostate, bronchus), myelomatosis, abscess, visceral referred pain, anatomical defects such as *spondylolisthesis* (forward slipping of a vertebra on the one below) or HLA-B27-related spondylitis (p 19). As a screening test an ESR is obligatory. For the rest, the history and physical examination should point to which tests are indicated. If a local lesion is suspected, but X-rays are negative, a bone-seeking isotope scan can be helpful. X-rays can be useful, but tend to be over-used. They are expensive and 'invasive' (irradiation to gonads, bone marrow, etc.). With careful clinical evaluation and an ESR, X-rays can be reserved for those patients in whom there is a pointer to some condition which may be revealed by radiology. In the absence of this it is reasonable to wait until backache has persisted for three months before ordering X-rays. The radiological changes are discussed on page 70 (Fig 7.2). Contrast myelography, involving the injection of radio-opaque dye, is reserved for cases in which surgical intervention is contemplated, or when other lesions are suspected.

The *prognosis* is unpredictable. Severe radiological spondylosis is compatible with no more than a few twinges of discomfort after unusual activity. However, patients with symptomatic lumbar spondylosis tend to run relapsing courses of recurrent backache with or without sciatica.

Treatment is often unsatisfactory. Acute exacerbations are treated in the same way as acute lumbar disc lesions (p 74). Surgical intervention is required less often than for acute disc lesions (apart from spinal stenosis—*see below*). The indications for myelography are the same as in the case of acute disc lesions (p 74). Some patients find that recurrences can be prevented or aborted by wearing a *lumbar (Goldthwaite) belt*. All patients should be instructed in *back care*, including the proper method of lifting. *Manipulation* is widely used in the treatment of disc and spondylotic disease at both the cervical and lumbar level. This ranges from manipulation under anaesthesia by the orthopaedic surgeon, through various grades of 'osteopathic' manipulations, to relatively gentle mobilisations by physiotherapists. No satisfactory controlled clinical assessment of these techniques has ever been achieved. The strongest evidence for the value of manipulation (albeit anecdotal) is the testimony of those whose acutely 'locked' backs have been dramatically relieved by manipulation. There is less evidence for the value of manipulation in chronic low back (or neck) pain. Nevertheless, this complaint is often so intractable that most chronic sufferers are given manipulation at some stage. If this is done, it is essential to ensure there is no evidence of an alternative lesion, such as a secondary deposit. Also, manipulation should be undertaken only with great care in anyone with a neurological deficit. If manipulation does relieve pain, it is not known how it achieves this.

Lumbar spinal stenosis

Lumbar spondylosis may produce bony encroachment on the spinal canal, with compression of the contents. The initial size and shape of the canal may determine how likely this is to occur. The history is often characteristic: a middle-aged man with a previous history of a disc lesion and sciatica, begins to experience his sciatic pain again. However, now the pain has a somewhat claudicant element, coming on with walking and easing slowly on sitting or lying. Weakness and numbness of the legs may also occur. Cauda equina ischaemia can be confirmed by either contrast myelography or by computerised axial tomography. If the symptoms are severe enough to justify it, surgical decompression (laminectomy) can provide relief.

8 Metabolic deposition arthritis: crystal synovitis

There are three joint diseases known to result from deposition of a metabolic produce in the articular tissues:

Disease	Metabolite	Joints involved
Gout	Urate	Peripheral small joints
Pyrophosphate arthropathy	Calcium pyrophosphate dihydrate	Large limb joints
Ochronosis (alkaptunuria)	Homogentisic acid metabolites	Central (spinal) joints

All three may lead to chronic destructive changes in the joints involved, but urate and pyrophosphate may in addition provoke episodic attacks of acute arthritis thought to be due to presence of microcrystals within the synovial fluid: *crystal synovitis*.

Crystal synovitis
During an attack of acute gout or pyrophosphate arthropathy ('pseudogout') polarised light microscopy shows the synovial fluid to contain large numbers of polymorphonuclear leucocytes, many of which contain microcrystals. There is strong experimental evidence that it is the interaction of these polymorphs and the crystals which results in the release of inflammatory substances. The precipitating events are unclear but, once the crystals are in the synovial fluid they become coated with protein, including IgG. Activation of complement follows, attracting polymorphs into the fluid, and these phagocytose the crystals. The process of phagocytosis itself releases inflammatory mediators, and the subsequent death of the polymorph (due to the presence of ingested crystals) releases lysosomal enzymes and other inflammatory substances. After a few days the (untreated) attack subsides—also for reasons which are not clear. Colchicine, which is more or less specific in aborting the acute gouty attacks, has no effect on urate metabolism, but is thought to act by interfering with polymorph function.

Other types of crystal may also be inflammatory within joints. The occasional acute reaction following intra-articular injection of corticosteroid probably depends on the same mechanism.

Hydroxyapatite crystals

Crystals of hydroxyapatite (the mineral in bone) are too small to see by polarised light microscopy. They have, however, been identified by electron microscopy in the synovial fluid of some cases of osteoarthritis, and there is speculation that they may possibly account for inflammatory episodes in that disease (p 63).

Hydroxyapatite is the substance most often laid down when soft tissue calcification occurs, for example in systemic sclerosis (p 39) and dermatomyositis (p 50). In these circumstances it does not cause inflammation. However, when it is laid down near the shoulder joint in calcific supraspinatus tendinitis (p 102) it can provoke acute inflammation, perhaps in a manner analogous to crystal synovitis in joints.

Gout

Gout is an arthropathy caused by the deposition of urate in and around joints. It results from a sustained elevation of uric acid in the plasma (hyperuricaemia). 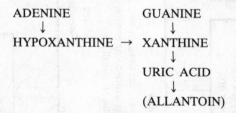 *Can get normocaemic gout*

Purine metabolism and hyperuricaemia

Uric acid is a divalent weak organic acid. In (acid) urine it exists as free uric acid, in tissue deposits as monosodium urate. It is produced as the end product of purine metabolism according to the following (simplified) scheme:

$$
\begin{array}{ccc}
\text{ADENINE} & & \text{GUANINE} \\
\downarrow & & \downarrow \\
\text{HYPOXANTHINE} & \rightarrow & \text{XANTHINE} \\
& & \downarrow \\
& & \text{URIC ACID} \\
& & \downarrow \\
& & \text{(ALLANTOIN)}
\end{array}
$$

The final stage takes place in lower animals, but not in man, who has suffered an apparently disadvantageous mutation resulting in loss of the enzyme *uricase*, and leaving uric acid as the end product of purine metabolism.

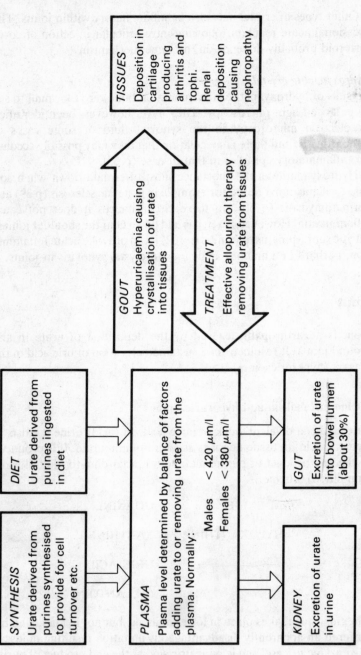

Figure 8.1 Factors determining the level of urate in plasma and deposition in the tissues

Renal handling of urate. Urate is freely filtered, then completely reabsorbed from the proximal tubule, a proportion being resecreted into the urine more distally. (The process is complex and not fully understood. Some post-secretory reabsorption probably also occurs.) This bidirectional tubular transport is an active process, shared by other weak organic acids such as aspirin. This accounts for the fact that the net effect of aspirin in small doses is to cause urate retention, while larger doses produce urate elimination.

Aetiology of hyperuricaemia

The plasma urate level depends on the factors shown in Fig 8.1. About one-third of elimination is into the gut. Purine synthesis varies with the rate of cell turnover, and is thus greatly increased in conditions such as leukaemia. The rate of renal excretion is markedly influenced by drugs such as thiazide diuretics, which produce hyperuricaemia and, if continued for sufficiently long, may cause gout.

Normally the balance of factors shown in Fig 8.1 results in a level of urate in the plasma which in males does not exceed about 420μmol/litre or 380μmol/litre in females. Blood samples for testing need to be taken fasting and off drugs such as aspirin and diuretics. These are arbitrary cut-off levels. A proportion of normal (non-gouty) people have higher levels.

The disease gout occurs when, because of elevation of the level in the plasma, urate is precipitated out into the tissues (Fig 8.1). The level at which this occurs is not all that far removed from the physiological level, and a variety of factors may contribute to the hyperuricaemia which leads to gout. Consideration of Fig 8.1 shows that hyperuricaemia may result from either excessive synthesis or reduced elimination of urate. Hence gouty patients are subdivided into *overproducers* or *underexcretors*. The distinction requires determination of the 24-hour urinary urate output which, on a low purine diet, should not exceed 3.6 mmol. A further subdivision is into *primary* (when no cause can be found) or *secondary* (when hyperuricaemia results from a factor such as overproduction, as in leukaemia, or underexcretion, as in chronic thiazide administration). These terms are oversimplification. *Most gout is multifactorial.*

Many other factors are known to influence the plasma level of urate. Changing from a normal to a low *dietary purine intake* can reduce the plasma levels by about 50 μmol/litre. Dietary purines and *alcohol consumption* (which acts in a variety of ways metabolically as well as by adding dietary purines) probably explain why gout was previously a rich man's disease. The action of drugs on the renal handling of urate has been mentioned. The ketoacidosis of *diabetes*, *starvation* and *glycogen storage disease* also cause urate retention. *Lead nephropathy*, e.g. from contaminated illicit alcohol, is another cause ('Saturnine gout'). *Hypercalcaemia* and *myxoedema* also act at a renal level. *Psoriasis* may be associated with hyperuricaemia, possibly through increased cell turnover in the skin.

When hyperuricaemia leads to urate deposition in the tissues the favoured sites are cartilage, particularly hyaline articular cartilage and the pinna of the ear, and the renal parenchyma. Why the cartilage particularly of small peripheral joints is selected by urate is unknown. It is likely that hyperuricaemia has been present for many years by the time clinical gout appears.

Clinical features

About 90 per cent of gout sufferers are men, about half give a positive family history and the onset is in the fourth to sixth decade.

The disease usually presents as a monarticular attack of crystal synovitis which settles in a week or two to leave a completely normal joint. Further similar attacks may follow at intervals of weeks, months or years. Some never experience more than one or two attacks. In others repeated attacks occur, and after a time the joints no longer return to normal between attacks. Deposits of urate become clinically apparent as *tophi* around joints and on the pinna of the ear. The final picture may be one of chronic deforming polyarthritis with periodic subacute exacerbations in one or a few joints— *chronic tophaceous gout*. *Renal impairment* appears in a proportion of long-standing cases, and a few patients pass urinary urate calculi (*urate urolithiasis*).

The first attack commonly affects the metatarsophalangeal joint of the great toe—*podogra*. Subsequent attacks may return to the same joint, to the opposite side, or elsewhere, but proximal joints such as the hip and shoulder tend to be spared.

The attack is often dramatically acute. Pain and swelling increase over a few hours until the joint is tensely swollen, red, hot, and exquisitely tender.

Sometimes malaise, fever and raised ESR reflect a systemic reaction. Untreated, the attack may last for days or weeks. Acute attacks may be precipitated by trauma, illness, operation or excess alcohol. Plasma uric acid levels are not particularly high during attacks and, surprisingly, sudden *lowering* of the level (as when drug

why ear + foot
? local pH/Temp
⇒ ppt of urate

Metabolic deposition arthritis **83**

therapy is started) is a potent precipitating cause. The mechanism of this is unknown.

Chronic tophaceous gout results when tophaceous deposits destroy the articular surfaces and lead to secondary degenerative changes in many, particularly peripheral, joints. *Tophi* appear as firm nodules attached to joints or on the helix of the ear. They may also occur in bursae or tendons, sometimes elsewhere. Tophi may soften and discharge chalky urate.

Renal disease may take the form of urate calculi (in about 20 per cent) or of intrinsic renal disease. Urate calculi are radiolucent on abdominal X-rays. Their formation is favoured by a concentrated, highly acid urine.

Many chronic tophaceous gout subjects show evidence of renal dysfunction (proteinuria, raised blood urea or hypertension). This presumably results from parenchymal urate crystal deposits and the resulting cellular reaction. But the issue is clouded by the association of gout and hypertension (*see below*), and the fact that renal disease may itself cause hyperuricaemia.

Secondary gout results either from overproduction of urate or underelimination by the kidneys. The checklist of conditions which have to be considered include:

Increased purine turnover	*Decreased renal urate excretion*
Myeloproliferative disorders (myeloid leukaemia, polycythaema vera, myelosclerosis)	Primary renal disease
	Drugs (thiazide diuretics, pyrazinamide etc.)
Other leukaemias	Hypercalcaemia
Other neoplasms	Myxoedema
	Glycogen storage disease
	Lead nephropathy

Associated diseases. Amongst gouty subjects there is an increased prevalence of *hypertension, diabetes, ischaemic heart disease* and *raised serum triglyceride* levels. The significance of this is not clear. There is no evidence that therapeutic reduction of the plasma urate level influences the other conditions.

Investigations

The essential investigations are determination of the *plasma uric acid* level (p 81) and the identification of urate crystals in synovial fluid or tophi by *polarised light microscopy* (p 135). Measurement of the 24-hour urinary urate output (p. 81) may also be useful.

Appropriate investigations will be needed to exclude the various causes of secondary gout (*see above*).

X-rays are normal early in the disease. Later they show bony 'erosions' at the sites where tophi have invaded bone. This occurs only at a stage of the disease when tophi are already obvious clinically. This radiological sign thus has little diagnostic value (in contrast to the erosions of rheumatoid arthritis). Long-standing tophi may show secondary calcification.

Diagnosis

An absolutely firm diagnosis requires identification of urate crystals in synovial fluid, other articular tissues, or in material from a tophus. Polarised light microscopy makes this simple provided appropriate material is obtained. If this diagnosis is in doubt, every effort should be made to obtain synovial fluid during an attack.

In the absence of crystal identification a reasonably confident diagnosis can be made if a man with a positive family history and elevated plasma level of urate develops typical podagra. A tophus clinches it, but this usually appears late. A persistently normal level of urate in the plasma of a patient not on a urate-lowering drug makes a diagnosis of gout highly unlikely.

In the absence of a typical history it is unwise to equate the association of joint pains and hyperuricaemia with gout. In these circumstances it becomes essential to obtain synovial fluid for crystal examination. From another point of view, no case of unexplained arthritis has been fully investigated unless fluid from an involved joint has been examined for crystals.

Acute gouty arthritis has to be differentiated from acute infection (septic arthritis or overlying cellulitis), from palindromic rheumatism (p 113) and from pseudogout (p 87).

Once a diagnosis has been made, it is necessary to consider whether any of the factors listed on page 83 as causes of 'secondary' gout may be operating. A drug history will tell whether the patient has been taking a thiazide diuretic, for example, while splenomegaly may be the clue to a myeloproliferative disorder.

Treatment

Treatment of gout involves two separate issues: firstly, termination of the acute gouty attack once it has started and, secondly, prevention of further attacks and continued tissue deposition of urate.

Acute gouty arthritis

The acute gouty attack is treated by prompt administration of an anti-inflammatory drug in large doses. Time-honoured colchicine (1 mg at once, then 0.5 mg 2-hourly until the attack subsides) may cause diarrhoea, and for this reason has mainly been replaced by indomethacin (50 mg four times daily), phenylbutazone (200 mg four times daily), or naproxen (250 mg four times daily). These doses are reduced progressively over a few days as the attack subsides. Having decided which drug suits him best, the patient should keep a supply of this on hand to start at the earliest warning of further attacks.

If a joint is aspirated for diagnostic purposes the opportunity can be taken to inject corticosteroid.

If the patient is already taking a urate-lowering drug such as allopurinol, this should be continued during the attack. However, *allopurinol and other urate-lowering drugs should never be started during an acute attack*. They may worsen and prolong the attack.

Long-term management

Once the acute attack has been controlled it is necessary to consider whether long-term management is needed.

The mildest cases may require no drug treatment. A single attack of acute gout in a patient with mild hyperuricaemia is an indication to review all the factors which may be contributing to this (diet, alcohol intake, obesity, drugs, etc.) and to advise the patient accordingly. Infrequent attacks in a mildly hyperuricaemic patient may be controlled by a small regular dose of colchicine (0.5 mg once or twice daily).

Urate-lowering drugs are indicated in the following circumstances:

Tophaceous gout
Frequent acute attacks
Gout with renal damage
Gout with plasma urate levels above 480 μmol/litre

The first choice amongst urate-lowering drugs is allopurinol, the second is the uricosuric agents.

Allopurinol competitively inhibits the enzyme *xanthene oxidase*, which brings about the conversions of hypoxanthine to xanthine and the latter to uric acid (p 79), and also suppresses purine biosynthesis. Its administration brings about a rapid fall in both plasma and urinary urate levels.

The daily dose of allopurinol required to bring the plasma urate levels to normal is 100 to 400 mg. However, rapid lowering of the level tends to provoke acute attacks (p 82). For this reason the drug is usually started in a dose of 100 mg daily (with concurrent colchicine 0.5 mg twice daily or another non-steroidal anti-inflammatory drug) and the dose gradually increased until the plasma urate level is normal. At that point the colchicine can be stopped. Once started, allopurinol should be continued indefinitely. Maintenance of a normal plasma urate level should not only prevent acute attacks, but also withdraw the urate which has been deposited in the tissues (Fig 8.1). In addition, by lowering urinary urate levels, allopurinol prevents stone formation.

Uricosuric drugs block renal tubular reabsorption of uric acid, thus increasing urinary urate output. The choice lies between probenecid, ethebenecid (both 0.5 to 1.0 g twice daily) and sulphinpyrazone (100 mg three or four times daily). These drugs are less effective than allopurinol, particularly in those with renal damage, and they may actually increase the risk of stone formation. They are used when allopurinol is not tolerated or, occasionally, together with allopurinol to get an added effect.

The *prognosis* for gouty subjects has been greatly improved by the introduction of effective urate-lowering drugs, particularly allopurinol. Provided the drug is tolerated it should be possible to achieve complete and permanent disease control.

Lesch-Nyhan syndrome

This excessively rare X-linked disorder is of interest as an example of a single enzyme defect causing gout. Affected male infants exhibit spasticity, choreoathetotic movements, mental deficiency and compulsive self-mutilation (biting the fingers and lips). Plasma and urinary urate levels are high and may result in gouty arthritis, uric acid stone formation and tophi. The syndrome results from a deficiency of hypoxanthine guanine phosphoribosyl transferase (HGPRT), the absence of which alters purine intermediate metabolism and causes overproduction of urate.

Other rare inborn errors of metabolism may be associated with hyperuricaemia.

Pyrophosphate arthropathy (pseudogout: chondrocalcinosis)

Like gout, pyrophosphate arthropathy results from the deposition of a crystalline metabolite in joint tissues. The cause of calcium pyrophosphate dihydrate (CPPD) deposition is unknown. The deposits are visible on X-rays as *chondrocalcinosis*. They may cause attacks of acute crystal synovitis—*pseudogout*—or chronic degenerative joint changes. However, the deposits are often asymptomatic.

Aetiology and pathogenesis

Minor deposits of CPPD in joint cartilage are extremely common in old age and are often asymptomatic. This age-related tendency for pyrophosphate to be laid down can presumably be exaggerated by a variety of different factors to produce heavier deposition—and resulting joint disease—at a younger age. A genetic factor must operate in the familial cases, while some metabolic factor presumably accounts for CPPD deposition in diseases such as hyperparathyroidism. In the majority of 'primary' cases no factor is discovered. The relationship with osteoarthritis is a matter for speculation. There is good evidence, on the one hand, that CPPD deposits can cause degenerative changes while, on the other hand, cartilage damage may predispose to CPPD deposition. This 'chicken and egg' problem is unsolved.

When CPPD deposits produce arthritis, this may take the form of episodic acute crystal synovitis (p 78), the crystals presumably entering the synovial fluid from deposits in cartilage, or chronic degenerative changes. In the latter case the crystalline deposits may alter the physicochemical state of the joint cartilage and interfere with its function as a bearing.

Clinical features

In *familial pyrophosphate arthropathy* (such as certain Czechoslovakian families) joint symptoms first appear in early adult life. In the much more common non-familial cases pyrophosphate arthropathy is usually first diagnosed in the middle-aged or elderly. It lacks the male preponderance of classical gout.

Much radiological chondrocalcinosis—particularly in the elderly—is asymptomatic. When arthropathy occurs it may consist of synovitis, chronic degenerative changes without acute attacks, or a mixture of acute episodes and chronic changes. Rarely subacute polyarthritis may mimic rheumatoid arthritis.

The acute attack

Pseudogout differs from acute classical gout attacks in generally involving larger joints and being somewhat less acute (in classical gout too attacks in larger joints may be less acute). Podagra has been described, but 'the knee joint is to pseudogout what the big toe is to gout'. Acute attacks may be precipitated by surgical operations, other illnesses, or by taking diuretics. A common presentation is for one knee to become swollen and painful while the patient is in a surgical or medical ward for some other reason. Attacks affect one or a few joints and, untreated, usually last for a week or two; but they may grumble on subacutely for a number of weeks. The affected knee is warm, often with reddening of the overlying skin. There may be a systemic disturbance with fever and leucocytosis—circumstances which are easily mistaken for septic arthritis if the synovial fluid is not examined for crystals and the tell-tale chondrocalcinosis not seen on X-ray.

Chronic degenerative arthritis

Degenerative changes associated with CPPD deposition occur mainly in the larger limb joints such as the knee and the shoulder. The clinical picture can resemble that in primary osteoarthritis, or there may in addition be superadded episodes of crystal synovitis.

The observation that chondrocalcinosis sometimes occurs in patients with the familial 'primary' type of osteoarthritis (with Heberden's nodes—p 64), and sometimes in neuropathic (Charcot) joints (p 113) suggests that degenerative joint changes may themselves predispose to CPPD deposition, so the relationship between CPPD and osteoarthritis may be complex.

Associated conditions

Most patients with pyrophosphate arthropathy do not have evidence of a metabolic disorder. However, there does appear to be an association with hyperparathyroidism, haemochromatosis, hypophosphatasia and classical (urate) gout; possibly also with acromegaly, Wilson's disease and diabetes. The reason for these associations is unknown. The presence of CPPD in Charcot joints has been mentioned above.

At the wrist CPPD deposits may be associated with *median nerve compression* (carpal tunnel syndrome—p 105).

Investigations

Examination of synovial fluid for crystals. This is described on page 135.

It is the most positive means of establishing the diagnosis. Specimens should be submitted in a plain sterile container without anticoagulant.

Polarised light microscopy can also identify CPPD crystals in synovial membrane biopsy material (absolute alcohol should be used as fixative).

Radiology. Chondrocalcinosis appears as a line of opacity in both hyaline articular cartilage and in fibrocartilage (knee menisci, glenoid and acetabular labra, symphysis pubis).

Much the most common site is the knee, after that the wrist (triangular ligament), hip, shoulder, symphysis, elbow and finger joints.

Rarely acute CPPD crystal synovitis may occur in a joint not showing chondrocalcinosis and, predictably, chondrocalcinosis may disappear when degenerative changes produce cartilage loss.

Other investigations may be indicated to exclude conditions such as hyperparathyroidism (p 88).

Treatment

Acute crystal synovitis is most effectively treated by *aspiration of the effusion* and *injection of corticosteroid*. Because larger joints are involved—particularly the knee—this method of treatment is more often applicable than in classical gouty attacks.

Non-steroidal anti-inflammatory drugs are employed, as in the gouty attack (p 85) but the value of colchicine is uncertain.

Ochronosis (alkaptonuria)

In this extremely rare autosomal recessive disorder the enzyme *homogentisic acid oxidase* is missing, so the degradation of tyrosine is blocked and homogentisic acid accumulates. The urine darkens on standing and pigmented metabolites accumulate in cartilage, giving the ears a slate blue appearance.

Deposition in the intervertebral discs produces spondylotic changes, sometimes with gross spinal rigidity and deformity. Proximal limb joints are occasionally involved. X-rays show disc space narrowing, spondylosis and secondary calcification.

9 Infective arthritis

The relationship of microbial infections and rheumatic diseases is complex. At one end of the scale is the relatively straightforward situation in which bacteria (e.g. staphylococci or tubercle bacilli) invade the joint tissues to produce local inflammation and destruction. At the other end of the scale 'inflammatory arthropathies' such as rheumatoid arthritis may possibly result from a particular pattern of immunological response to a microbial infection in a genetically susceptible individual (p 3). Between these two extremes fall 'reactive arthritis' (p 20) in which polyarthritis follows a more clearly defined microbial infection—without invasion of the joint by the organism. Finally, in certain cases of Neisserial and virus infections the organism can be isolated from the joint, but polyarthritis appears to result, not from local multiplication and invasion by the organism, but from a systemic immunological reaction. Such 'postinfective arthritis' may follow meningococcal, hepatitis B or rubella infections. Dumonde has proposed the classification shown in Table 9.1 to illustrate current concepts about these associations of infection and arthritis.

This chapter is concerned mainly with Types 1 and 2 in Table 9.1. Page references in the Table indicate where other infection/arthritis associations are mentioned.

Acute suppurative arthritis

Septic arthritis may be apparently 'primary', in which case it affects mainly children, or it may occur secondary to some other local or systemic condition. Most infections are due to staphylococci or streptococci, but almost any organism may be involved.

Routes of infection

Childhood infections usually reach the joint either via the blood stream, sometimes from an identifiable distant focus such as otitis media, or directly from an adjacent bone infection. Penetrating wounds or intra-articular injections may also introduce infection.

Table 9.1 A suggested classification for the associations between infection and arthritis (after Dumonde).

Type	Microbial infection known	Presence or multiplication of organisms in joint	Presence of microbial antigen in joint	Designation of arthritis, syndrome or association	Illustrative examples
1	Yes	Yes	Yes	'Infective'	Suppurative (septic) (p 90) Tuberculous (p 94)
2	Yes	Presence inconsistent. Probably no local multiplication	Yes	'Postinfective'	Postmeningococcal arthritis (p 94) Arthritis associated with hepatitis B (p 96), and (?) rubella (p 95)
3	Yes	No	No	'Reactive' (p 20)	Rheumatic fever (p 97) Yersinia arthritis (p 20)
4	Suspected but unproven	No	No	'Inflammatory'	Rheumatoid arthritis (p 3); SLE (p 33).

Secondary septic infection is a rare but definite complication of rheumatoid arthritis. The presence of any foreign body in a joint predisposes to infection, and secondary infection remains one of the important complications of prosthetic joint replacement.

Pathology

Initially there is synovial hyperaemia, polymorph infiltration and serous effusion. Later the effusion turns purulent, the cartilage becomes softened, and granulation tissue grows into the synovial cavity. Untreated, the result can range from spontaneous resolution to destruction of the joint and death from septicaemia. The outcome depends on the virulence of the organism and the resistance of the individual. Antibiotic treatment can cut short the process.

Clinical features

In the most acute cases the patient is febrile and toxic, and the joint distended with fluid, warm with overlying erythema, spontaneously painful, extremely tender, and movements are almost impossible because of pain. The joint tends to be fixed by muscle spasm in the position in which the capsule is least under strain (for example partial flexion of the hip or knee joint).

In less acute cases the clinical features may be much less dramatic. Corticosteroids may almost completely mask the signs.

Investigations

The ESR and white blood cell count reflect the acuteness of the infection. Blood cultures may grow the responsible organism. The synovial fluid can be serous or purulent, with total counts of about 50×10^9/litre and, of these, over 95 per cent are likely to be polymorphs. However, a low cell count does not exclude infection (and a turbid fluid may occasionally occur in an uninfected rheumatoid or crystal synovitis joint). A stained smear may reveal the organism, but culture is of course mandatory. Chemical methods of identifying organisms are being tested. Gas-liquid chromatography reveals high levels of lactic acid in infected joint fluids.

X-rays are normal in the early stages. Later there may be osteoporosis and loss of 'joint space'.

Diagnosis

Many arthropathies can occasionally present a sufficiently acute picture to raise the possibility of infection. *The safe rule is always to aspirate such joints for bacteriological investigation*. Crystals should be looked for at the same time (p 135). Superadded infection in a rheumatoid joint can cause confusion; but again, if in doubt, aspirate. Patients on steroids may show greatly reduced inflammatory reaction to pyogenic arthritis.

Treatment
The affected joint should be immobilised by bed rest, splinting or traction. Analgesics will be needed.

Drainage is achieved by daily aspiration so long as the effusion reaccumulates. If loculation occurs surgical drainage may be needed.

Antibiotics are started as soon as specimens of synovial fluid and blood have been obtained for bacteriological examination. Antibiotics readily enter the infected joint. Intra-articular administration is therefore employed only when the joint is needled for other purposes. Antibiotics should be continued for some weeks after the inflammation settles. Failing precise bacteriological identification and sensitivity tests, the following guidelines may be used:

> *Presumed staphylococcal:* Flucloxacillin or clindamycin (in children under 3 years add ampicillin because of the possibility of *H influenzae*).

> *Pseudomonas and other Gram-negative rods:* Gentamycin with carbenecillin.

Prognosis
Provided treatment is started before irreversible damage has occurred, the outcome is usually satisfactory. Some residual secondary osteoarthritis is common.

Gonococcal arthritis

Gonococcal arthritis is seen mainly in females (presumably because the genital infection—less dramatic than in the male—is neglected). Presentation is often in association with menstruation or pregnancy.
   The presentation may be that of purulent arthritis in a single joint, but more often the patient experiences a migrating subacute polyarthritis and tenosynovitis, sometimes associated with features of septicaemia: papular skin lesions which progress to pustular or haemorrhagic vesicles, rarely meningitis or endocarditis. Gonococci

can usually be cultured from the joint fluid, and the response of the arthritis to penicillin is rapid.

Meningococcal arthritis

Like gonococcal arthritis, meningococcal arthritis may be purulent and involve one joint, or there may be migratory polyarthritis associated with the septicaemic phase. Organisms are inconsistently grown from involved joints. It may be that an immune complex ('serum sickness') type of reaction is involved.

Tuberculous arthritis

Tuberculosis of joints is always secondary to a focus elsewhere. The joint and adjacent bone are often affected simultaneously.

Clinical features
Children and young adults particularly are affected, and racial groups from the Indian subcontinent appear to be especially susceptible. In children the hip and knee joints are most commonly affected, in adults the vertebral column (Pott's disease).

General malaise, night sweats and loss of weight are common. One or a few joints are involved with features of subacute inflammation. Swelling and loss of function may be more prominent than pain. Spinal tuberculosis (Pott's disease) commonly involves the dorsal region. There is local tenderness and limitation of spinal movements. Once a vertebra collapses there may be a spinal angulation ('gibbus'). Occasionally tuberculous pus may track from the lesion to a distant site as a 'cold abscess'.

Investigations
The ESR is generally raised and the Mantoux test positive. To establish the diagnosis material must be obtained for bacteriological identification, or at least histology, from within the joint. Failing that, a therapeutic trial may have to be undertaken.

X-rays can be normal in the early stages, or there may be a lucent area in bone indicating a periarticular bone abscess. Later there is loss of 'joint space' and marked rarefaction. In the spine (Fig 9.1) there may be collapse of one or more vertebral bodies with *loss of related intervertebral disc spaces* (an important sign in differentiating

infective from malignant lesions). The faint fusiform outline of a
spinal abscess may be visible.

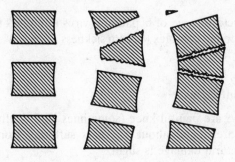

Figure 9.1 In bacterial infections of the spine, adjacent disc spaces tend to be
involved together with the vertebral body (*right*). By contrast, malignant
involvement (*centre*) spares the discs. Diagram of normal X-ray appearance
on left

Treatment

Until the result of sensitivity tests becomes available the patient is
usually started on rifampicin, isonazid and ethambutol. The joint is
rested, if necessary by splinting. In many instances surgical intervention is undertaken to drain an abscess, excise a focus in bone, or to
perform a synovectomy. It also provides material for histological and
bacteriological examination (including sensitivity). In the spine surgical fusion may be undertaken.

Viral infections

A variety of viral infections may occasionally be complicated
by arthritis. Rubella is the most common type, occurring
particularly in young adult females, but arthritis may also complicate
mumps, infectious mononucleosis, smallpox and chicken pox. A few
or many joints may be involved. Usually there is spontaneous
resolution within six weeks, but occasional cases of rubella arthritis
have persisted for over a year and come to resemble rheumatoid
arthritis. Rubella arthritis may appear before, during or after the
rash, or occasionally without any rash. The diagnosis then depends
on a history of exposure, typical peripheral blood changes, and rising
antibody titres. Carpal tunnel syndrome and tenosynovitis are not
uncommon complications. Histological changes are inconspicuous.
The virus can sometimes be isolated from the synovial fluid. Treat-

ment is symptomatic. A short course of corticosteroids is sometimes employed to cut short the arthritis. Arthritis may also follow rubella vaccination.

In the pre-icteric stage of hepatitis B virus infections there may be a transient immune complex ('serum sickness') phase with polyarthritis and urticaria.

Spirochaetal infections

Clutton's joints are painful knee (sometimes elbow) effusions which occur in children aged about 12 years suffering from congenital syphilis. Structural damage is slight.

Secondary syphilis may also produce transient knee effusions.

Fungal infections

A wide variety of fungi may occasionally infect joints. Often this is secondary to spread from an adjacent bone focus. Fungal infections are more common amongst patients with debilitating diseases or suppressed immunity. The clinical differentiation from tuberculosis may be impossible without culture of the fungus.

10 Rheumatic fever

(a touch of Rheumatism)

This inflammatory disease affects children and young adults. It follows streptococcal pharyngitis and the chief features are polyarthritis, carditis and chorea. It has become rare in affluent societies.

Incidence

for

Over the past 35 years in countries such as the United Kingdom rheumatic fever has changed from a common and important disease to a rarity. This may relate to the influence of factors such as housing on the epidemiology of streptococcal infections. Rheumatic fever is still common in parts of the Middle East and Africa. Children between 6 and 15 years are most often affected.

Aetiology

triggered by virus or bacterial / trauma etc.

Rheumatic fever appears to be an example of 'reactive arthritis' (pp 20 and 90). Previous infection with a group A beta-haemolytic streptococcus sets off a reaction pattern which is presumed to be immunologically mediated. There is some evidence for antigenic cross-reactivity between cardiac tissue and the streptococcal cell wall.

Clinical features

migratory polyarthritis

The disease usually presents with *polyarthritis* about three weeks after a streptococcal sore throat. Multiple joints are generally affected, particularly larger limb joints, and the pattern of involvement is characteristically *flitting*, each joint being involved for a few days at a time. Affected joints are hot, red, swollen and extremely painful. Histological changes are generally unimpressive, and permanent damage does not occur (except in the rare curiosity known as *Jaccoud's syndrome*—p 113). *Fever* is a constant feature and parallels disease activity.

Carditis of some degree occurs in 50 per cent of initial attacks in children. It is less common in adults. The typical histological finding is a granuloma, the *Ashoff body*. All layers of the heart may be involved. *Myocarditis* produces tachycardia and sometimes dysrhythmias or even cardiac failure. *Endocarditis (valvulitis)* produces soft cardiac murmurs during the acute stage. The apical mid-diastolic ('*Carey Coombs*') murmur indicates active mitral valvulitis. The mitral valve is most commonly affected, next the aortic. Regurgitation or stenosis of these valves may develop gradually over months or years, sometimes to be recognised only later in life. *Pericarditis* may present as chest pain with a pericardial friction rub, or as a pericardial effusion. If carditis occurs during the initial attack, recurrent attacks are likely to cause increasing permanent valvular damage. If no carditis occurs in the first attack, subsequent attacks are unlikely to involve the heart.

Sydenham's chorea may occur as the only manifestation of rheumatic fever, or it may accompany other features. It is more common in females. Chorea is characterised by abnormal purposeless jerking or writhing movements of the limbs and facial grimacing. Items are dropped unintentionally and difficulty is experienced in writing and doing up buttons etc. Emotional lability often accompanies these movements, which are occasionally unilateral (*hemichorea*). They cease during sleep. Chorea is self-limiting, subsiding after a period of weeks or months.

Erythema marginatum is the characteristic skin manifestation of rheumatic fever, occurring in about 10 per cent of cases. The lesion is a transient pink macule with pale centre and darker margin which creeps outwards irregularly to cover expanding, irregular areas, sometimes coalescing with other lesions.

Subcutaneous nodules occur in less than 10 per cent of cases. The shotty, painless subcutaneous nodules are found over pressure points, particularly the occiput and extensor surfaces of joints. Histologically they consist of central fibrinoid necrosis surrounded by a variety of inflammatory cells, including multinucleated giant cells. The differentiation from rheumatoid subcutaneous nodules can be difficult.

Abdominal pain may occasionally be the presenting symptom.

Investigations
Disease activity is reflected by elevation of the *ESR* and *C-reactive protein*. *Mild anaemia* and *polymorphonuclear leucocytosis* are common. *Throat swabs* in the early stages may grow haemolytic strepto-

cocci. Later a raised or rising titre of *Antistreptolysin O* (ASO) antibodies indicates a recent streptococcal infection. Titres of 1/500 ('500 units') or greater are significant.

Course

Rheumatic fever occurs in attacks which may last from a few weeks to many months. Without prophylaxis recurrences are common—usually triggered by further streptococcal infections. They become both less common and also less liable to involve carditis after the age of 18 years.

Diagnosis

A great many diseases of childhood enter into the differential diagnosis of rheumatic fever. The diagnostic weight to be attached to various features is reflected in the *Jones criteria:*

Major criteria	*Minor criteria*
Polyarthritis	Fever
Carditis	Arthralgia
Chorea	Prolonged PR interval
Erythema marginatum	Raised ESR
Subcutaneous nodules	Previous rheumatic fever or established rheumatic heart disease.

Two major, or one major plus two minor criteria are considered strongly suggestive of rheumatic fever, especially with evidence of preceding streptococcal infection.

Juvenile chronic polyarthritis tends to differ from rheumatic fever in that smaller, more peripheral joints may be involved in a more sustained (not 'flitting') manner and the local inflammation is usually less acute. Also, rheumatic fever is rare below the age of 5 years.

Treatment

Strict *bed rest* is traditional, but its value is unproven.

Both *salicylates* and *corticosteroids* will suppress the inflammatory features (particularly the arthritis) but there is no evidence that they affect the final outcome. Soluble aspirin dosage (100 mg/kg body weight per day in divided doses) is adjusted according to clinical response and blood levels (between 20 and 25 mg/100 ml). *Prednisolone* (2 mg/kg body weight per day) is reserved for the most severe cases such as those with cardiac failure or pericarditis.

Antibiotics do not affect the course of an attack of rheumatic fever, once started, but a course of penicillin is usually administered whether or not streptococci are grown on throat swab. *Prophylactic antibiotic therapy* to prevent recurrences is highly effective. Oral phenoxymethyl penicillin 125 to 250 mg twice daily is usually employed, or monthly injections of a long-acting penicillin. Prophylaxis is continued for five years or until the subject is an adult, whichever is longer. In patients with established valvular disease dental procedures should be 'covered' with antibiotics to prevent bacterial endocarditis.

Prognosis

Very few patients die during the initial acute attack. The prognosis for permanent valve damage is proportional to the signs of carditis in the initial attack. Overall about 50 per cent develop some permanent valve changes. Occasional patients present with apparent rheumatic valvular lesions for the first time in adult life without ever having suffered from clinically obvious rheumatic fever or chorea.

11 Medical orthopaedics ('soft tissue rheumatism')

Collected into this chapter is a variety of conditions affecting the soft tissues of the locomotor system. None is primarily arthritic. Although relatively minor, most of these conditions are important because they are common and treatable.

Shoulder lesions

The stability of the shallow shoulder joint is maintained largely by the 'rotator cuff', consisting of the incorporation into the capsule of flattened expansions of the tendons of subscapularis and supraspinatus anteriorly, and infraspinatus and teres minor posteriorly. In addition, the long head of biceps holds the humeral head into the glenoid cavity. Immediately above the joint, and often communicating with it, lies the *subacromial bursa*.

This anatomical arrangement may account for the frequency with which the shoulder is affected by a variety of ill-understood disorders in which pain and stiffness are the outstanding features. The most likely factor appears to be mechanical trauma leading to a cycle of pain, immobility and stiffness; but the pathology is not understood.

Nor is it known to what extent these conditions are separate entities or variations on a single theme. The traditional descriptive terms used below imply an exactness of anatomical and pathological diagnosis that is often not justified.

'Rotator cuff lesions'

The most common pattern of painful shoulder is that in which pain is provoked by the execution against resistance of a movement brought about by one of the rotator cuff muscles. What at first may appear to be a generally painful and stiff shoulder can, on careful examination, prove to have a relatively free and painless range of motion, except for one particular movement, the execution of which (especially against resistance) produces pain. This finding is regarded as evidence of 'tendinitis' of the muscle tendon in question. Examples of tendinitis include:

Tendon	Painful resisted movement
Supraspinatus	Abduction
Infraspinatus	External rotation
Subscapularis	Internal rotation
Biceps	Supination and flexion of elbow.

Occasionally what starts as an isolated tendinitis may apparently spread to involve the whole rotator cuff, with pain on all resisted movements, and this is then referred to as '*capsulitis*'. If very gross limitation of all passive movements at the glenohumeral joint develops, then the descriptive term '*frozen shoulder*' is applied. However, this evolution from one pattern of shoulder problem to another is less common than for the patient to present with 'tendinitis', 'capsulitis' or 'frozen shoulder' from the beginning, and for this pattern then to persist.

Rotator cuff lesions occur in young or middle-aged adults. The onset may be spontaneous or may follow a strain or injury. Passive shoulder movements are reasonably full, but when movements served by the involved tendon are attempted against resistance a sharp pain is produced. Pressure over the site of the tendon insertion may reproduce the pain, which can range from mild to very severe. It lasts for weeks or months, then always recovers completely.

Supraspinatus tendinitis is the most common rotator cuff lesion. Following a minor strain or trauma, spontaneous pain appears, usually referred (as in other shoulder lesions) to the point of insertion of the deltoid muscle. Examination reveals tenderness over the greater tuberosity. Passive shoulder movements are often reasonably full, but active abduction of the arm reveals the typical *painful arc* sign. That is, pain through the intermediate range of abduction (60° to 120°). Characteristically the 'painful arc' pain is lessened by external rotation of the arm. Resisted abduction produces sharp pain. X-rays may show *supraspinatus tendon calcification*. This X-ray appearance is occasionally associated with spontaneous attacks of severe local pain. These possibly represent attacks of acute *crystal synovitis* (p 79) from softening and rupture of the calcific material into the tendon sheath or joint cavity.

Calcification in a tendon suggests a degenerative process. However, occasional patients exhibit calcification besides multiple joints (*multiple calcific periarthritis*). These can produce repeated acute inflammatory episodes. The relationship of this generalised disorder to isolated supraspinatus tendinitis is unclear.

Treatment of rotator cuff lesions. The first line of treatment is a local injection of corticosteroid (e.g. 50 mg of hydrocortisone acetate—with or without preliminary local anaesthetic) into the region of the affected tendon or, in the case of more general capsulitis, into the subacromial bursa. This can be dramatically effective. However, if one or more injections do not relieve the pain it is customary to prescribe exercise and heat, etc. The value of these measures is unproven. Eventual complete recovery can in any case be confidently predicted, but this may take many months.

Bicipital tendinitis. Pain on elbow flexion and forearm supination against resistance, combined with tenderness anteriorly over the bicipital groove indicates *bicipital tendinitis*. Treatment is by local corticosteroid injection. In very obstinate cases surgical immobilisation will eliminate pain without affecting function.

Subacromial bursitis
Because of its situation, this bursa is probably frequently involved in rotator cuff lesions. Occasionally it may become distended with fluid to bulge out from beneath the acromion. A needle passed under the acromion readily enters the bursa and, unless a more specific target is sought, this is a satisfactory site for injecting corticosteroids for painful shoulders. Whether this bursa becomes inflamed as a primary event is uncertain.

Frozen shoulder (adhesive capsulitis)
This is a more serious condition, occurring in an older age group. Various grades of restriction may occur with other painful shoulder conditions, but 'frozen shoulder' refers to almost complete loss of all glenohumeral movements. The pathological changes include tight contraction of the joint capsule.

The condition may arise spontaneously, or follow trauma, or occur with conditions which produce pain and/or immobility in the arm: hemiplegia, herpes zoster, breast operations, etc. It may also apparently be provoked by ischaemic heart disease or pulmonary lesions.

Pain, especially at night, can be extremely severe and distressing. Gradually over the months it eases to leave mainly stiffness. The condition eventually improves spontaneously and, after a period of about 18 months, the patient is left with a somewhat restricted, but painless, shoulder.

Probably the best treatment is prophylactic. Mobilisation of the shoulder in patients with hemiplegia or other neurological lesions, or breast surgery, may well prevent the shoulder becoming 'frozen'. The established condition is very resistant to treatment. Local corticosteroid injections give little relief, and physiotherapy is of unproven value. Mobilisation under anaesthesia combined with prednisolone by mouth is currently being tested. Analgesics and the application of local heat at night (by electric pad) may be needed over a long period.

Shoulder-hand syndrome
This is a rare condition in which a frozen shoulder becomes associated with swelling, stiffness and pain in the hand on the same side. The same aetiological factors appear to operate. It is extremely incapacitating. The swollen hand shows vasomotor and trophic changes. It is held immobile and protected in a manner reminiscent of causalgia. X-rays of the hand show patchy osteoporosis suggestive of Sudeck's atrophy. Physiotherapy, corticosteroids and cervical sympathectomy have been advocated for this condition, but no treatment is reliably effective. At least partial improvement occurs after months or years.

Tennis elbow (lateral humeral epicondylitis)

This extremely common condition occurs mainly in young and middle-aged adults. Pain develops gradually over the outer aspect of one elbow. Sharp exacerbations may occur on executing particular manoeuvres. Examination reveals a joint which is normal, except for localised tenderness over the lateral epicondyle (the exact tender point may be difficult to locate) and the pain is reproduced by forceful contraction of the muscles which arise from the lateral epicondyle, for example dorsiflexion of the wrist against resistance.

The pathology is unknown. As in the case of plantar fasciitis (p 107) it is assumed to be a response at the fibro-osseous junction to some mechanical factor. Untreated the condition waxes and wanes, then settles spontaneously after a period of weeks or months. It can usually be cured by a local injection of local anaesthetic followed by 50 mg of hydrocortisone acetate into the site of maximum tenderness. Some patients find that firm strapping over the upper forearm is effective. A variety of surgical procedures are effective, but rarely required.

Golfer's elbow (medial humeral epicondylitis)

This (less common) condition is exactly comparable to tennis elbow, but affects the inner (medial) elbow epicondyle. Resisted wrist flexion provokes the pain. Treatment is the same, but injection techniques must take account of the nearby ulnar nerve.

Nerve entrapment: carpal tunnel syndrome

Certain peripheral nerves are particularly vulnerable to compression by the structures through which they pass. Well known sites for this are the *lateral popliteal nerve* as it winds round the neck of the fibula, and the *ulnar nerve* at the elbow. However, much the most common nerve entrapment involves compression of the median nerve at the wrist: *carpal tunnel syndrome*. The bones of the wrist form a concavity on the palmar surface, which is roofed over by the flexor retinaculum. Through this 'tunnel' pass the flexor tendons in their sheaths, and the median nerve. Any swelling of the contents may compress the nerve.

Carpal tunnel syndrome occurs in adults of all ages, more commonly in women. It can arise spontaneously, but it also occurs in association with a wide variety of general (sometimes local) disorders, the common factor being an increase in the bulk of the contents of the canal. Predisposing conditions include obesity, pregnancy, myxoedema, acromegaly (p 108) and rheumatoid arthritis (p 7). Carpal tunnel syndrome is extremely common amongst rheumatoid patients. In them the diagnosis can easily be overlooked because both patient and doctor ascribe pain and muscle wasting to the joint disease. This is a serious error, for the compensated function achieved in the damaged rheumatoid hand is particularly vulnerable to a superadded neurological deficit.

The patient will often give a characteristic history. She is woken at night by a painful, numb, tingling sensation in the hand and seeks relief by hanging the arm out of the bed and wringing the hand. These symptoms are often diffuse and not accurately localised to the distribution of the median nerve. Fine finger function may be impaired.

In mild cases there are often no abnormal physical signs, or perhaps tapping over the middle of the wrist joint anteriorly may cause tingling in the distribution of the median nerve (*Tinel's sign*). In more severe cases there may be altered sensation in the palmar aspect of the radial $3\frac{1}{2}$ digits and wasting and weakness of the thenar muscles (*Opponens pollicis* is tested by getting the patient to pinch the tips of the thumb and little fingers together; *abductor pollicis brevis* moves the thumb from a position beside the palm, forwards at right angles to the palm). Electrical tests may show impaired nerve conduction, but this test is sometimes normal in mild cases.

Treatment is highly effective. Mild cases are either given a wrist splint to wear at night, or the carpal tunnel is infiltrated with 0.25 ml of a soluble corticosteroid preparation. In resistant cases, or those with an obvious neurological deficit, the flexor retinaculum is divided surgically. Underlying causes may require attention.

De Quervain's syndrome (tenosynovitis of abductor pollicis longus)

The long abductor of the thumb forms the anterior border of the anatomical snuff box. Tenosynovitis may develop at the point where it crosses the radial styloid process. Pain is often poorly localised, but extension of the thumb in abduction reproduces the pain, and this is aggravated if the examiner exerts pressure on the tendon during this manoeuvre. Infiltration of the sheath with corticosteroid is usually effective. Failing this, immobilisation of the thumb by splinting, or surgical release of the tendon sheath is necessary.

Trigger finger (stenosing tenovaginitis)

In this minor disorder a thickening on a finger flexor tendon tends to stick as it passes through a narrowed segment of its sheath. Either flexion or extension of the digit may be affected: movement proceeds freely up to a point, then the finger sticks. Exerting greater force eventually overcomes the resistance and the movement is completed with a snap. The site of stenosis is usually opposite the metacarpo-phalangeal joint. Local injection of corticosteroid into the tendon sheath is usually effective. Failing that, surgical relief of the constriction is simple and curative.

Achilles' tendinitis

Pain and swelling may occur around the point of insertion of the Achilles' tendon into the calcaneal bone. This probably usually represents an inflammatory reaction at the fibro-osseous junction ('enthesopathy', as in plantar fasciitis—*see below*) but there may also be an associated *bursitis*. Sometimes there is an obvious cause, such as pressure from an ill-fitting shoe or a mechanical strain of some sort. Often no cause is apparent. Achilles' tendinitis may also occur as a feature of a *seronegative spondarthritis* (p 19) such as ankylosing spondylitis or Reiter's disease, in which case it may represent part of the general tendency to periosteal new bone formation, especially over bony prominences. Treatment is by injection of local anaesthetic followed by corticosteroid. Footwear may require adjustment.

Plantar fasciitis (painful heel)

Pain on the undersurface of the heel on weight bearing is an extremely common complaint. Like Achilles' tendinitis (*see above*) it appears to be an 'enthesopathy', the inflamed fibro-osseous junction in this case being the posterior attachment of the plantar fascia to the calcaneum. It may represent a form of foot strain, or it may occur as a manifestation of a seronegative spondarthropathy (p 19). Pain is reproduced by pressing the thumb firmly upwards into the centre of the heel.

X-rays may show a protruding spur of bone at the painful site. This is smooth in the case of 'simple' plantar fasciitis, but fluffy and eroded in cases of seronegative spondarthropathy. Treatment is by injection of local anaesthetic followed by corticosteroid down to the periosteum at the painful site (pain may be considerably aggravated over the following 18 hours).

Morton's metatarsalgia

This refers to pain in the forefoot radiating to the adjacent sides of the third and fourth toes caused by an interdigital neuroma. Treatment is by a metatarsal insole pad or excision of the neuroma.

The rheumatological importance of this condition is that it can easily be mimicked by early rheumatoid arthritis affecting the metatarsophalangeal joints.

12 Less common rheumatic and related conditions

The disorders listed alphabetically in this chapter include uncommon arthropathies and general diseases which occasionally have rheumatic features.

Acromegaly

Excess growth hormone produces overgrowth of connective tissue. Articular cartilage shares in this and the radiological 'joint space' becomes widened. There is also excessive new bone formation. Clinically, these patients may present with degenerative changes in peripheral and spinal joints. *Carpal tunnel syndrome* p 105) is common, and *chondrocalcinosis* p 87) may occur.

Amyloidosis

Amyloidosis may complicate rheumatoid arthritis (p 10) or any of the other systemic connective tissue diseases (p 32). It may cause carpal tunnel syndrome (p 105). Rarely, amyloidosis secondary to myelomatosis may infiltrate joints to present as polyarthritis.

Anaphylactoid (Henoch-Schönlein) purpura

This is a rare form of vasculitis affecting particularly young children, and manifesting as polyarthritis, purpura, abdominal pain and nephritis. It sometimes follows a streptococcal infection, but usually no precipitating event is identified. The circumstances suggest a serum-sickness type of pathogenesis (p 115), but this has not been proven. Autoantibodies are not a feature.

The *arthritis* consists of transient synovitis affecting a few joints. The typical *skin lesion* appears on the legs and buttocks as a raised papule (cf. thrombocytopenic purpura) with a purpuric spot at the centre. *Abdominal pain* is occasionally accompanied by *gut haemorrhage* or *intussusception*. *Proliferative glomerulonephritis* occurs in up to half these patients. Occasionally it becomes progressive. Corticosteroids may be of value in cases with serious gut involvement.

Aseptic (avascular) necrosis

The head of the femur appears to be particularly vulnerable to infarction and collapse of a segment of bone at the upper (weight-bearing) pole. Less commonly other joints are involved. The condition may arise for no obvious cause, or it may complicate an inflammatory polyarthritis. It may also complicate a wide variety of other circumstances, including corticosteroid therapy (especially for renal transplantation), caisson (decompression) sickness, alcoholism, haemoglobinopathies, femoral neck fracture, etc.

Typically there is a sudden onset of pain in one hip, and the joint becomes irritable and restricted. X-rays are normal at first, but the isotope scan (p 136) shows a 'hot' joint. Later X-rays show a depressed quadrant of bone at the upper pole, although the 'joint space' (cartilage) is well preserved. Various degrees of remodelling and secondary osteoarthritis result. Weight-bearing should be avoided in the early stages. Later surgical joint replacement may be indicated.

Behçet's syndrome

It is not certain whether this constitutes a single disease entity. The diagnosis is usually based on the association of *mouth, genital* and *skin ulcers* with *inflammatory eye lesions*, particularly *iritis*. However, a very wide variety of other features have been described, including inflammatory polyarthritis, serious central nervous system lesions, thrombophlebitis, gastrointestinal, cardiovascular and pulmonary lesions, etc.

Treatment is symptomatic unless uveitis (particularly with hypopyon) threatens sight or serious CNS features are present, in which case corticosteroids and immunosuppressive drugs are tried.

Chondromalacia patellae

In late teenagers and young adults a painful condition may develop in the patellofemoral compartment of one or both knees. The pathogenesis is unknown. The more severe cases eventually develop 'degenerative' changes in the cartilage over the posterior patellar surface and medial femoral condyle. The patient, often an athletic girl, complains of intermittent aching and sometimes slight swelling of the knee. Examination reveals a normal main knee compartment, but pressure over the patella during contraction of the quadricips ('press your knee down on to the couch') is sharply painful. The posterior surface of the patella may be tender. Effusions are uncommon.

Treatment is symptomatic. Reduction of activity, occasionally splinting, analgesics, heat, quadriceps exercises, even corticosteroid injections are tried, although their value is unproven. A variety of operative procedures, such as shaving the patellar cartilage, have also been advocated. Fortunately, the condition tends eventually to settle spontaneously.

Erythema nodosum

Erythema nodosum is a type of cutaneous vasculitis in which painful, tender erythematous nodules appear, particularly down the front of the shins. After a few days they take on the colour of a bruise.

Erythema nodosum appears to be a reaction pattern which may be triggered by such diverse conditions as sarcoidosis (p 114), inflammatory bowel disease (p 31) and leprosy, or it may occur without obvious cause.

Whatever the trigger, erythema nodosum tends to be accompanied by malaise, fever, raised ESR and, in a proportion of cases, *polyarthritis*. The knees and ankles are most often involved. The joints settle without residua within days or weeks. Treatment is symptomatic.

Familial Mediterranean fever

Familial Mediterranean fever is inherited as an *autosomal recessive gene*, mainly among *Sephardic Jews* originating in the Eastern Mediterranean.

The condition usually presents in the second decade with intermittent episodes of *high fever* and *serositis*, including *abdominal and pleural pain*, and *synovitis*. The synovitis is usually monarticular, particularly in a knee. The often very acute arthritis usually settles over a few days to leave an undamaged joint. Later, degenerative changes may appear. Fatal *amyloidosis* is a common complication.

Haemochromatosis (iron overload arthropathy)

Arthritis occurs in about half the patients with haemochromatosis. Typically, this presents as degenerative changes in metacarpophalangeal and proximal interphalangeal joints, but episodic synovitis of larger joints may also occur. More than one mechanism may be involved. A proportion of these patients have radiological *chondrocalcinosis* (p 87), so pyrophosphate deposition and crystal synovitis may be involved. In addition, iron overload from other causes (*transfusion siderosis, sideroblastic anaemia*, etc.) may also be associated with arthritis, and iron is deposited in the joints. However, the mechanism by which iron deposition causes the arthritis is unknown. Correction of iron overload does not improve the joints.

Haemoglobinopathies

Haemoglobinopathies, particularly homozygous *sickle-cell disease*, may cause a variety of osteoarticular complaints. *Bone infarcts, haemorrhages into bones and joints* and *remodelling of bones* due to erythoid hyperplasia may produce bone and joint pains. *Aseptic necrosis* (p 109) and *septic arthritis* (p 90) are other complications.

Haemophilia

In most boys with either haemophilia or Christmas disease recurrent bleeds into joints are a major problem.

Acute haemarthrosis may occur spontaneously or follow minor trauma. The affected joint becomes swollen, hot and extremely painful. Treatment is by full intravenous replacement of the missing factor VIII or IX at the first warning of a bleed. This may require home treatment.

If tense, the effusion should be aspirated (after replacement therapy). Analgesics will be needed. The knee is rested in a splint while acutely painful, then subsequently mobilised (with muscle-strengthening exercises) under adequate replacement therapy.

Recurrent bleeds into a joint can eventually produce a chronic, boggy synovium with cartilage and bone destruction, looking not unlike rheumatoid arthritis, and particularly liable to further bleeds. Such joints occasionally justify surgical debridement, arthrodesis or arthroplasty, although the replacement therapy requirements are daunting.

Hypermobility syndromes

There is considerable variation between individuals in the range of movement that is normal. In general, greater mobility is seen in the young, in females and in pigmented races. Clinical evidence of hypermobility includes the ability to perform some of the following:

Hyperextend the little finger to 90°.
With wrist flexed, place the thumb against the forearm.
Hyperextend the knee and/or elbow beyond 10°.
Standing with knees straight, place the palms on the floor.

Gross hypermobility with joint and ligamentous laxity is a feature of certain inherited disorders of connective tissue (Ehlers-Danlos and Marfan's syndromes). Lesser degrees of hypermobility tend to run in families, and these may be associated with a tendency to dislocate the shoulders or patellae, and also with a variety of joint problems: backache, arthralgia, secondary osteoarthritis and chondrocalcinosis (p 87).

Hyperparathyroidism

Hyperparathyroidism may produce joint disease in different ways: secondary gout (p 81), chondrocalcinosis and pyrophosphate arthropathy (p 87) and joint changes secondary to underlying metabolic bone disease.

Hypertrophic (pulmonary) osteoarthropathy

Severe finger clubbing from any cause may be associated with a peripheral arthritis affecting particularly the wrist and ankle. There is pain, tenderness, swelling, and the overlying skin may be warm, red and oedematous. X-rays show characteristic *periosteal new bone formation* round bones adjacent to affected joints.

Bronchial carcinoma is by far the commonest cause. Resection of the primary lesion, or simply section of the vagus nerve may relieve the symptoms.

A very rare primary form is *pachydermo-periostosis* (Touraine-Solente-Gole syndrome).

Hypogammaglobulinaemia

Severe congenital or acquired hypogammaglobulinaemia is sometimes associated with polyarthritis which resembles mild rheumatoid arthritis. It is benign, non-erosive and seronegative.

Jaccoud's syndrome

The arthritis of rheumatic fever (p 97) normally leaves no residua. Rarely, after numerous severe attacks, there may develop mild permanent deformities. These are due to soft tissue fibrosis rather than synovitis, and include flexion and ulnar deviation at the metacarpophalangeal joints, and sometimes 'hook-like' erosions of the metacarpal heads.

Leukaemia

Both acute and chronic leukaemia can produce joint symptoms either by synovial infiltration or by involvement of bones adjacent to joints. Childhood leukaemia may present with a picture mimicking inflammatory polyarthritis.

Neuropathic (charcot) joints

Loss of pain sensation from a joint makes it vulnerable to progressive destructive changes. The classic example is the Charcot joint of tabes dorsalis, but similar changes may occur in syringomyelia, diabetic neuropathy or other causes of loss of pain sensation. Any joint may be involved, including the spinal joints, and the features are those of gross osteoarthritis, progressing to disorganisation and destruction of the joint. Physical examination reveals gross crepitus or even subluxation in a painless joint. Neuropathic joints in diabetic feet are exceptional. These may be painful and mimic infective lesions.

Osteochondritis dissecans

In this condition flakes of articular cartilage become separated to form loose bodies within the joint. The flakes remain alive (nourished by synovial fluid) and frequently ossify. This commonly affects one knee in a teenager or a young adult, and presents with features of a loose body (locking, giving way and recurrent effusion). If the cartilage flake carries away a piece of underlying bone with it the defect may be visible on X-ray. Treatment is by surgical removal of the loose body.

Palindromic rheumatism

One of the more dramatically acute forms of arthritis is palindromic rheumatism, in which recurrent episodes of joint inflammation last a few hours or days, then resolve to leave a normal joint. Adults of any age may be affected. Usually one joint is involved in an attack. Sometimes the sites involved are away from joints, producing oedema, erythema or nodules in the skin. Attacks may continue for many years at intervals of days, weeks or months, without change. However, at some stage about 50 per cent of cases evolve into otherwise typical *rheumatoid arthritis* (p 3). It remains unclear whether palindromic rheumatism is a separate condition which may trigger rheumatoid arthritis, or whether the two are variations on a single theme.

The acute attack is treated with non-steroidal anti-inflammatory drugs. Interval treatment with gold injections (p 12) has been suggested.

Pigmented villo-nodular synovitis

This rare condition affects the synovium of a joint or a tendon sheath in a young adult. It presents as a synovial effusion which, on aspiration, is deeply blood-stained.

In long-standing cases destructive bone changes occur. The lesion is a villous or nodular overgrowth of synovium with giant cells and haemosiderin. It is unclear whether it is neoplastic, haemangiomatous or inflammatory in nature. Treatment is by synovectomy, sometimes combined with irradiation. Recurrences are common.

Relapsing polychondritis

If this extremely rare disease affecting the middle-aged there occur recurrent episodes of inflammation involving cartilage. Clinically there may be polyarthritis and inflammation and collapse of the cartilage of the ears, nose and tracheal rings, the latter being an important cause of death. An autoimmune reaction against cartilage probably underlies the lesions. Corticosteroids may damp down individual episodes, but the long-term prognosis is poor.

Sarcoidosis

Two types of arthritis may occur in sarcoidosis. The first is a benign and relatively common form seen particularly in young women. Sometimes referred to as *Löfgren's syndrome*, it consists of a triad of *erythema nodosum* (p 110), radiological *hilar adenopathy* and *polyarthritis*. Complete recovery occurs within weeks.

The *granulomatous* type is rare and more serious. Granulomata develop in the synovium and produce progressive chronic changes with deformity which may mimic rheumatoid arthritis. It usually occurs with multisystem sarcoidosis and carries a poor prognosis.

Serum sickness

Characteristically serum sickness follows about seven days after a therapeutic injection of foreign (horse) serum. This represents the time interval needed for the patient to produce antibodies to the foreign serum proteins and for these to reach the critical level (slight antigen excess) at which soluble immune complexes are formed. These activate the complement system and produce widespread vascular damage. Clinically there is *urticaria, lymphadenopathy, fever, proteinuria* and *polyarthritis*.

Nowadays foreign serum is seldom given therapeutically, but serum sickness remains the classical model of circulating immune complex disease. It may be mimicked, for example, in the pre-icteric phase of *hepatitis B virus infection* (p 96). In this case the circulating virus acts as the provoking antigen. Similarly, the nephritis and arthralgia sometimes complicating *bacterial endocarditis* are probably mediated by circulating immune complexes provoked by bacterial antigens. Another example is the acute arthritis of *lepromatous leprosy*. Here again bacterial antigens can be detected in the circulating immune complexes. During active serum sickness serum complement levels fall through consumption.

Synovial (osteo) chondromatosis

Metaplasia of joint synovium may occasionally lead to the formation of multiple nodules of cartilage. These tend to become pedunculated or actually separate as loose bodies nourished by the synovial fluid. They frequently become calcified or ossified. The multiple opacities present a dramatic picture on X-ray.

A knee is usually affected, and these loose bodies predictably tend to produce locking and giving way of the joint, followed by periods of swelling. Treatment is by surgical removal of the loose bodies.

Synovial rupture

A knee joint effusion produces very high intra-articular pressures during flexion under load. This may lead to posterior rupture of the joint cavity with tracking down of the fluid into the calf. The physical signs are then almost indistinguishable from those of a deep calf vein thrombosis, including a positive Homans' sign (calf pain on dorsiflexing the ankle). Spontaneous resolution usually occurs over days or weeks, but occasionally a calf cyst forms. The diagnosis may be confirmed by arthrography, when the injected radio-opaque dye will be seen to track into the calf. The rheumatoid knee is the joint which ruptures most commonly, but effusions from any cause may rupture, and joints other than the knee are sometimes involved.

Synovial tumours

Malignant tumours of joints are rare. *Secondary metastases* may occasionally involve joints.

Malignant synovioma arises from synovial cells. It is a very rare and highly malignant tumour of adults. It usually presents as a painless swelling beside, rather than within, a joint.

Whipple's disease

Polyarthritis is one feature of this rare disease in which there is also *steatorrhoea, wasting* and *pigmentation*. The small intestinal lymph nodes contain periodic-acid-Schiff positive material in macrophages, and the condition responds to tetracycline treatment (suggesting a pathogenic role for some bacterial agent).

Appendix A **History taking**

Informed history taking provides as much diagnostic information as do the physical examination and investigations. The cardinal symptoms of joint disease are pain, stiffness, swelling and loss of function.

Pain

Lay concepts about 'rheumatism' can distort patients' descriptions of pains which they believe are due to joint disease. Thus the first objective may be to decide whether pain actually arises in the joints. Particular hazards are painful skeletal disorders such as metabolic bone disease and multiple myelomatosis, both of which can produce 'rheumatic' types of pain.

Peripheral limb joint pain is easier. It may be accompanied by other local evidence of arthritis—particularly swelling—and be provoked by movement of the articulation in question. Also, it is usually well localised to the joint from which it arises. However, an important exception to this is the hip: pain arising here may be felt (sometimes exclusively) in the knee joint on that side (referred via the obturator nerve which supplies articular branches to both joints). Shoulder joint pain may be felt at the point of insertion of the deltoid.

In mild osteoarthritis pain may occur only as mild twinges on executing particular movements. However, advanced osteoarthritis of the hip or knee can interfere with sleep through pain at night, and the pain of a 'frozen shoulder' is usually most troublesome at night. Gout, septic arthritis or a haemophilic bleed may produce constant severe pain which prevents all movement.

Neck, trunk and limb girdle pains can be confusing. In both the cervical and lumbar regions, spondylosis or disc lesions may cause local aches of wide distribution, which are often accompanied by referred (nerve root irritation) pain radiating into the limb. These pains tend to be aggravated by spinal movements, and the referred component may be provoked by manoeuvres which raise intraspinal pressure (sneezing and straining).

Sciatic pain closely related to exercise (claudicant) is suggestive of lumbar spinal canal stenosis. Ankylosing spondylitis tends to produce diffuse aching pains in the whole trunk and down the legs as far as the knees.

Neurological conditions may mimic arthritic pain. In carpal tunnel syndrome the nocturnal pain is relieved by hanging the hand down and shaking it. Pre-eruptive herpes zoster pain has a superficial smarting quality. Other hazards are Bornholm disease, neuralgic amyotrophy and the lightning pains of tabes dorsalis. By contrast, neuropathic (Charcot) joints are characteristically painless, except in the diabetic foot where they may be misleadingly painful (p 113).

Stiffness

Joint stiffness is an imprecise complaint, covering sensations which range from slight resistance to all movements through the normal range, to blocking of certain movements due to fixed anatomical changes. Many patients find it difficult to separate joint stiffness from pain—understandably, as both may arise from common factors such as capsular tension. Certain types of stiffness are highly characteristic.

Early morning stiffness occurs in rheumatoid arthritis, other inflammatory arthropathies (juvenile chronic arthritis and the seronegative spondarthropathies) and in polymyalgia rheumatica (p 47). The patient awakes with distressing, painful stiffness of all affected joints. This is gradually 'worked off' by activity over one half to three hours or more. This 'limbering up time' provides a reliable measure of inflammatory activity. Taking a hot bath can give some relief. The stiffness may reappear during the day if the patient spends a period sitting immobile. Patients with ankylosing spondylitis may be aware that physical activity lessens both pain and stiffness, while rest worsens both.

Lesser degrees of early morning stiffness may occur in conditions such as systemic lupus erythematosus, but in osteoarthritis stiffness tends to come on later in the day and to follow activity.

'Locking' refers to sudden blocking of some part of the normal range of movement. Together with *'giving way'* it is characteristic of interposition of something between the articulating surfaces. In the knee joint this symptom is suggestive of either a meniscal lesion or a loose body.

'Trigger finger' (p 106) is caused by a thickened segment of a finger flexor tendon having to pass through a narrowed section of its sheath.

Either flexion or extension of the digit sticks at a certain point. When greater effort is applied the movement is completed as a sudden jerk.

Swelling
A history of swelling of a joint is important as an indication of whether a patient has experienced actual arthritis. Pain in a joint without abnormal physical signs is referred to as 'arthralgia'. Patients are usually reliably aware of whether joints have been swollen.

A history of swelling (and/or redness) beside a joint, rather than over it, may be a pointer to palindromic rheumatism (p 113) or to an extra-articular lesion such as pre- or infrapatellar bursitis, or Achilles' tendinitis (p 106). The sudden appearance of a painful calf swelling may suggest a ruptured knee synovium (p 115).

Loss of function
Functional capacity (FC) can usefully be graded according to the following simple scheme:

Grade I	Completely independent without any adaptions
Grade II	Independent with some adaptions (e.g. aids and appliances)
Grade III	Partially dependent (e.g. needing help with bathing or dressing)
Grade IV	Confined to bed/wheelchair

Joint noises
Joint 'cracking'—as on hyperextension of a finger or full knee flexion under load—represents 'cavitation' (sudden formation of a gas bubble in the synovial fluid) and is of no pathological significance. Similarly, quite impressive crepitant sounds may be heard during normal scapular/shoulder movements. By contrast, creaking or 'klunking' noises arising from hip or knee joints while weight-bearing indicate significant structural damage. Coarse crepitus from roughened joint surfaces (p 64) may be audible to the patient and to others.

Pattern of joint involvement
The distribution of joint involvement as revealed by the history may be highly informative. Rheumatoid arthritis characteristically starts as a symmetrical peripheral small joint polyarthritis, while the seronegative spondarthropathies tend to be less symmetrical and to involve the spine. Gout usually affects peripheral joints, particularly

the first metatarsophalangeal (podagra), while the hip and shoulder are rarely involved. Pyrophosphate arthropathy generally affects larger limb joints, particularly the knee.

The wrist joints—so commonly involved in inflammatory arthropathies—are rarely affected by primary osteoarthritis. In the latter condition in middle-aged women, it is involvement of the thumb carpometacarpal joint and the terminal interphalangeal joints with Heberden's nodes which brings them to the doctor—often because they fear that they may have rheumatoid arthritis.

Extra-articular symptoms

In a patient suspected of suffering from a rheumatic disorder, history taking must clearly include interrogation about all other systems. However, there are certain features which have particular rheumatological significance. Diagnostic pointers may be provided by eye symptoms: conjunctivitis (Reiter's disease, p 28), iritis (ankylosing spondylitis, p 20), dry eye (Sjögren's syndrome, p 56, or scleritis (rheumatoid arthritis, p 8). Raynaud's phenomenon (episodes of numb white fingers, usually provoked by cold) may herald a systemic connective tissue disorder, while skin eruptions may provide important diagnostic clues: psoriasis (p 26), erythema nodosum (p 110), or the 'butterfly' rash of SLE (p 35). Important genital symptoms include urethritis (p 29), ulceration (p 30), penile psoriasis (p 27), and circinate balanitis (p 30). Recurrent mouth ulcers may suggest Behçet's syndrome (p 109), while inflammatory bowel disorders can be associated with the seronegative spondarthropathies (p 31).

A useful question to ask patients suffering from rheumatoid arthritis is 'Do you experience numbness or tingling of your hands or feet?'. The answer may provide a pointer to the recognition of an entrapment neuropathy (ulnar or median nerve, p 105), Raynaud's phenomenon (p 40), cervical myelopathy (p 72), or peripheral neuropathy (p 7).

Family history

Almost all rheumatological conditions show some familial clustering. Haemophilia is the most obvious example, but (apart from rarities) a positive family history may be an important lead also in gout, ankylosing spondylitis and psoriatic arthritis. It is of less value in rheumatoid arthritis and osteoarthritis.

Psychological and domestic factors

In anyone with a major rheumatological problem an attempt should be made to assess the overall impact of the disease on the patient and on his family. Obtaining information about attitudes towards disease, and judging the contribution of psychological factors to the patient's problems are clearly important—although beyond the scope of discussion in this chapter.

Other factors

It is necessary to establish whether the onset of joint symptoms was related to trauma; also, whether there is a relevant history of infection, or exposure to infection, including rubella, hepatitis, dysentery, tuberculosis or sexually acquired infections etc. Finally, information should be obtained about drug therapy.

Appendix B **Clinical examination of joints**

This section deals with the physical examination of joints. It does not attempt to cover general examination of the patient, nor the examination of other systems, although these are obviously required in patients with rheumatic diseases.

The locomotor system as a whole

Observation begins as the patient enters the room. Posture, gait, physique and deformities may provide valuable clues. It is particularly important to remember that the examination of a lower limb joint is incomplete until it has been studied while weight-bearing and during walking. An irritable hip may be missed in a fractious child on the couch, while the tell-tale limp will provide the clue to the site of the problem.

The individual joint

Paired joints should be examined together; each method of examination being applied simultaneously or alternately to the two sides for comparison. The minimum routine check involves *inspection*, particularly for swelling, *palpation*, particularly for tenderness, and *movement* of the joint through its full range. The complete examination of an individual joint should provide information about the following:

Swelling. In accessible joints swelling is usually apparent on inspection. However, palpation is necessary to differentiate three types:

Bony swelling of osteophytes in osteoarthritis
Synovial (soft tissue) swelling of inflammatory synovitis
Fluid (synovial effusion)

Osteophytes have a firm gnarled feel. Synovial swelling is soft and spongy, while fluid is also soft, but can be moved about the joint to give 'cross fluctuation' or other signs mentioned under individual joints. Also effusions may distend the joint into a characteristic contour.

More localised swellings may be encountered: ganglia (synovial herniations), deeper (Baker's) cysts, rheumatoid nodules or gouty tophi.

Overlying skin. Erythema of the overlying skin is an index of acuteness of joint inflammation. It is common in acute gout or septic arthritis, uncommon in the rheumatoid joint, and should not occur in osteoarthritis. A *rise in skin temperature* is a much more sensitive index of joint vascularity and is a surprisingly definite physical sign. One technique is for the examiner to test with the back of the fingers of one hand, moving backwards and forwards between the same skin area over the joint on each side of the body. By this technique some increased warmth is likely to be detected even over an osteoarthritic joint. Over the most acutely inflamed joints there may be *oedema* of the skin.

Tenderness generally reflects the acuteness of inflammation in a joint. However, accurate mapping of the tender area may give valuable information. Localised tenderness can indicate the site of a strain in an osteoarthritic joint (p 63), or may be the clue to a lesion outside the joint, such as pre- or infrapatellar bursitis, or De Quervain's syndrome at the wrist (p 106).

Range of movement

For routine examination of the spine and hands, *active* movements are generally studied, while for the remaining limb joints *passive* movements are usually more informative. In a diseased joint it may be helpful to test both types of movement. When the range of movement is abnormal it should be measured and recorded. The most useful measuring instrument is a protractor with hinged arms (*goniometer*). All movements are measured from the *zero starting position* in which the body is represented erect with hands by the sides, and toes, palms and nose pointing forwards (except for forearm movements which are measured from a zero starting position in which the elbow is flexed to 90° and thumbs pointing straight up). From these zero starting positions movements are recorded as degrees of flexion, extension, supination, pronation, etc. The range of normal movement varies considerably between individuals (*see* p 111).

Pain on movement

This is a reflection of irritability of a joint. In an osteoarthritic joint pain is often provoked only at the limits of the range. In an acutely inflamed joint any movement may be painful and resisted by muscle spasm.

Crepitus is a sensation of roughness or crunching transmitted from a moving joint to a palpating hand. It indicates roughening of the bearing surfaces. It is thus *fine* in the early stages of rheumatoid arthritis and *coarse* in advanced osteoarthritis (rough bone ends grating together). Tenosynovitis may produce *tendon sheath crepitus*.

Deformity. This term is—confusingly—used to describe three joint abnormalities. The first is inability to move through some part of the normal range, for example *flexion deformity* due to capsular contraction. The second is abnormal alignment of the bones, for example—in the knee—*valgus* ('knock knee') or *varus* ('bow leg') deformity. It is necessary to test whether such deformity can be corrected, and what the effect on it is of weight-bearing. The third type of deformity refers to altered relationship of the bearing surfaces: *subluxation* indicates that part of these surfaces still remain in contact, while *dislocation* implies complete loss of contact between these surfaces.

Stability. Defective bearing surfaces or lax ligaments may allow joint movements outside the normal range (e.g. valgus or varus movement in the knee). Such instability should be sought by passive movements designed to test integrity of the various ligaments (collapse of a bearing surface is an equally common cause of instability).

Muscles. In use, stability of joints depends largely on the pull of muscles acting across them. Joint disease leads to early weakness and wasting of these muscles (p 67). Hence assessment of muscle bulk and power is an important aspect of joint examination. In knee joint disease, measurement of thigh circumference at a specified distance above the top of the patella provides a useful comparison between the two sides. A rough estimate of quadriceps power may be made by pressing the tips of the fingers into the muscle while the patient forces his knee downwards on to the couch.

Functional tests. As well as individual joint movements it is necessary to test integrated functions such as *gait* and *grip*.

The spine

Adequate exposure is essential. Observe *posture* with the patient standing. Increased flexion is *kyphosis*, extension *lordosis*, and lateral bending *scoliosis*. A local lesion (infective, neoplastic or fracture) is suggested by angulation (*gibbus*) and local tenderness.

Assessment of movement requires correct positioning of patient and observer, and appropriate instructions to the patient.

In the notes that follow, the approximate average range of movement in healthy adults is indicated.

Cervical spine
The patient sits or stands.

Rotation (70°). 'Look over your shoulder to the left/right'.

Flexion (45°). 'Look down—chin on your chest'.

Extension (45°). 'Look up—tilt your head back'.

Lateral bending (45°). 'Bend your head to the left/right—ear towards your shoulder'.

Thoracolumbar spine
Rotational movements take place mainly at the thoracic level, bending movement in the lumbar spine region. Movements are assessed by eye. The patient is seated (to anchor the pelvis) when rotation is tested, but stands for the remaining tests.

Rotation. The seated patient, with arms folded across the chest, rotates the shoulders to the right/left.

Flexion. 'Touch your toes keeping your knees straight'. The lumbar spine is carefully observed during this manoeuvre. Normally the lumbar lordosis should convert to forward flexion. Rough documentation is obtained by measuring the increase in distance between two skin marks initially 10 cm apart over the lumbar spine (*Schober test*).

Extension. The patient leans over backwards, supported by the examiner's hand in the small of the back.

Lateral bending. 'Slide your right/left hand down the side of your leg so as to bend sideways, not forwards'.

Chest expansion. This useful measurement of costovertebral joint mobility is assessed by tape measure. Five centimetres is about the lower limit of normal, depending on build. It may be reduced early in ankylosing spondylitis.

Sacroiliac joints

The site of these joints is indicated by a pair of skin dimples. Pain on firm pressure with the thumbs at these points indicates sacroiliac irritability. The rigid bony ring of the pelvis makes it difficult to produce movement of the sacroiliac joints. One technique is to press firmly downwards over the centre of the pelvis with the patient prone. Another is to flex one hip fully while maintaining hyperextension of the opposite joint. Either manoeuvre will elicit pain in irritable sacroiliac joints.

Mandibular joints

A palpating finger placed just in front of the tragus of the ear will feel the head of the mandible sliding forwards as the jaw is opened. Tenderness, crepitus and clicking may be elicited. Incisor opening distance is a measure of the range of movement.

Shoulder girdle

Sternoclavicular and acromioclavicular joints

Both these articulations are easily inspected and palpated. Movements are tested by asking the patient to 'shrug the shoulders'.

The shoulder

Most shoulder movements are a combination of ball and socket motion at the glenohumeral articulation and sliding of the scapula over the rib cage. To test pure glenohumeral movement the scapula is anchored by the examiner placing a hand across the clavicle and scapular spine.

Painful/stiff shoulder conditions are discussed on pp 101–104. Attention is drawn there to the importance of testing for pain provoked by the execution of individual movements against resistance.

Abduction (glenohumeral 90°, total 180°). Glenohumeral abduction is tested passively, total elevation actively. Note that a rupture or paralysis of supraspinatus prevents *initiation* of abduction (deltoid can complete the movement). The *painful arc* is discussed on page 102.

Adduction (50°). The humerus is carried across the front of the chest.

Flexion (90°). Swing the arm forwards.

Extension (65°). Swing the arm backwards.

Internal rotation (90°). This is conveniently recorded as the distance the patient's thumb can reach up the back (a combined glenohumeral and scapular movement).

External rotation (60°). A pure glenohumeral movement. Usually tested with the upper arm by the side and the elbow flexed to 90°.

Elbow
The olecranon and proximal subcutaneous ulnar border should be examined for rheumatoid nodules, gouty tophi or a bursa. Medial and lateral humeral epicondylitis are described on pages 104–105.

Flexion (150°)

Extension (0°)

Forearm
The examiner's thumb placed 2 cm distal to the lateral humeral epicondyle will feel the head of the radius rotating within the annular ligament during passive supination/pronation at the forearm.

Pronation (90°). Rotate the wrist palm down.

Supination (90°). Rotate the wrist palm up.

Wrist
Primary osteoarthritis of the wrist is rare, so arthritis of this joint usually indicates an inflammatory condition, such as rheumatoid arthritis. However, *ununited fractures of the scaphoid, osteoarthritis of the first carpometacarpal joint* and *De Quervain's syndrome* (p 106) may all mimic wrist arthritis.

Flexion (75°)

Extension (75°)

Radial deviation (20°)

Ulnar deviation (30°)

Hand

Examination of the hand requires a good light and, ideally, patient and examiner should be seated opposite each other. The front and back of the two hands are examined first with fingers outstretched, then while the patient makes a fist. Not only the various joints, but the tendon sheaths and small muscles require attention too. Different types of arthritis produce characteristic changes in the hands, including 'nodular' osteoarthritis (Fig 6.2, p 66), rheumatoid arthritis (Fig 2.1, p 5 and psoriatic arthritis (p 26).

Lower limb

The hip

The depth of the hip joint from the surface makes it relatively inaccessible to direct examination. However, deep palpation over the centre of the inguinal ligament may elicit tenderness from an irritable joint. Examination of the hip begins with noting *posture* and *gait*. Three special tests may be useful:

Trendelenberg test. The examiner sits behind the standing patient and palpates the iliac crest on either side while the patient raises first one foot then the other off the floor. Normally the non-weight-bearing side rises upwards. With hip joint disease (or muscle weakness) it may sag downwards.

Concealed flexion deformity. The painful arthritic hip tends to be held in partial flexion (the position of least capsular tension). However, particularly in children, this may be concealed (compensated) by *exaggerated lumbar lordosis*. An effective test to reveal this is, with the patient lying supine, to flex the opposite hip forcefully. This abolishes lumbar lordosis (confirmed by the examiner's other hand in the small of the patient's back) and the knee on the affected side moves off the couch to reveal any hip flexion deformity.

Leg length. True leg length is measured from the anterior superior iliac spine to the medial malleolus, taking care that the two legs are in comparable positions in relationship to the pelvis. Reduction in true leg length may indicate destructive changes in the region of the hip joint. *Apparent leg length* is measured from umbilicus to medial malleolus. Difference not reflected in true length alterations imply pelvic tilt, usually due to an adduction deformity of one hip.

As with the shoulder joint (p 126) assessment of hip joint movements has to take account of the possibility that pelvic girdle movements may contribute to apparent hip joint movements. A hand placed on the iliac crest will detect such movement.

Flexion (115°). The flexed knee is pushed towards the chest.

Extension (30°). This awkward but important test may require an assistant. The patient lies on the opposite side, and the examiner extends the thigh, while keeping a hand on the iliac crest. The angle recorded is that at which further extension is achieved by pelvic tilting.

Abduction (50°). Pelvic movement must be checked.

Adduction (45°). The leg is carried across in front of the opposite limb.

Rotation (internal 45°, external 45°). This is usually tested with the hip and knee both flexed to 90°.

The knee
The knee should be examined both standing and lying, and the back of the joint must not be overlooked. The joint comprises two 'compartments', the patellofemoral and the main articulation.

Patellofemoral arthritis is revealed by pain and crepitus when the patient contracts the quadriceps ('force your knee down on the couch') while the examiner pushes the patella distally and backwards against the femur. Similarly pain may be elicited by rubbing the patella against the femoral condyles.

Synovial effusions. The synovial cavity extends upwards as the suprapatellar pouch. When the joint is distended with fluid this forms the upper part of a characteristic horseshoe-shaped swelling round the patella. Using both hands the examiner may elicit 'cross fluctuation' of the fluid. Less obvious effusions may be detected by special techniques. The *patellar tap* is performed by using the left hand to force fluid out of the suprapatellar pouch while the patella is pushed back against the femoral condyles by the fingers of the right hand. A distinct 'tap' as the patella meets the underlying femur is reliable evidence of an effusion. For smaller effusions the *bulge sign* is elicited by using the left hand both to compress the suprapatellar pouch and also (with the index finger) anchor the patella. The fingers of the right hand are then drawn along the groove between the patella and the femur—alternately on the medial and lateral sides. Small effusions may be detected by a bulging out of the groove as the opposite side is stroked.

Interpretation of physical signs in the knee requires consideration of the anatomy. The main joint is situated at the level of the middle of the patellar ligament and runs at right angles to the tibia. The head of the fibula is readily located, while the position of the two collateral ligaments can be estimated, and often confirmed by palpation. Careful palpation of the anteromedial and anterolateral aspects of the joint line during passive movement of the knee may reveal evidence of a meniscal cyst or tear. Anteriorly pre- and infrapatellar bursitis must be differentiated from arthritis of the knee.

Any *valgus* (knock-knee) or *varus* (bow-leg) deformity must be noted, both on the couch and while weight-bearing. In addition any *laxity* of the collateral or cruciate ligaments (instability) must be sought by attempting to move the extended knee into varus and valgus, and attempting anterior/posterior gliding movements of the tibia, both in extension and 90° of flexion.

Flexion (135°). Thigh and calf bulk may restrict this.

Extension (5°). A measure of 'hypermobility' (p 111).

Ankle
True ankle (mortise joint) lesions must be differentiated from *ligamentous strains* and adjacent tenosynovitis. Localise tenderness accurately. Test movements with the knee flexed.

Dorsiflexion (20°)

Plantar flexion (50°)

Foot
Not all the individual joints lend themselves to individual testing. Divide up the foot examination as follows:

Subtalar joint. Grip the lower leg with one hand while the other moves the heel passively from side to side (about 10° each way). Pain and limitation may indicate arthritis of this joint. View from behind the patient standing barefoot: *valgus* (*eversion*) deformity occurs in *pes planus* (flat foot).

Midtarsal joint. Grip the heel with one hand while twisting the forefoot into inversion and eversion. Note any flattening of the longitudinal arch while standing (*pes planus*).

The forefoot. Pinch each metatarsophalangeal joint and move it passively. Note thickening or irritability (an early sign of rheumatoid arthritis).

The toes. Apart from common deformities such as *hallux valgus* and *clawed toes*, the most informative sign is *interphalangeal joint arthritis* which occurs in the *seronegative spondarthropathies* (p 19).

Appendix C **Investigations**

Rheumatoid factors

Rheumatoid factors are antibodies (autoantibodies) directed against immunoglobulin G (IgG). They can be detected in most immunoglobulin classes, but the standard tests detect IgM rheumatoid factors. These are present in the serum of about 85 per cent of patients with rheumatoid arthritis—often in high titre, and occur in about 4 per cent of 'normals'—often in low titre. They may also be found in the serum of patients with other systemic connective tissue diseases (p 32), and certain other conditions (liver disease, bacterial endocarditis, etc.). Despite this 'overlap', and the fact that about 15 per cent of otherwise apparently typical rheumatoid arthritis patients remain seronegative throughout, tests for rheumatoid factors remain of fundamental importance in the diagnosis of rheumatoid arthritis. The two most commonly used tests are:

Latex flocculation test. Polystyrene particles are coated with human IgG and added to dilutions of serum. Flocculation at a dilution of 1/80 or greater is significant.

Sheep-cell tests (Rose-Waaler test). A variety of tests employ sheep erythrocytes lightly coated with rabbit IgG. This coating is achieved by exposing the red cells to subagglutinating dilutions of rabbit anti-sheep erythrocyte serum. The 'sensitised' sheep red cells are then added to dilutions of the patient's serum. Agglutination at 1/16 or greater is significant.

Of the two tests, the latex is easier to perform, more sensitive, but less specific.

LE cells and antinuclear antibodies

Autoantibodies to various nuclear antigens are characteristic of systemic lupus erythematosus, and may occur in other systemic connective tissue diseases (p 32). The laboratory tests used to detect them include:

LE-cell test

The LE cell is a phagocyte containing a mass of ingested nuclear material. The phenomenon occurs in two stages. First, antinuclear antibody attaches to the nucleus, then phagocytosis of the opsonised nucleus occurs. Peripheral blood leucocytes (prepared by some technique which introduces some mechanical trauma, thus allowing penetration of the cell membrane by antibody) are incubated, then stained and examined for LE cells.

The test is positive in about 80 per cent of patients with SLE, and may be positive also in chronic active hepatitis and other systemic connective tissue diseases (p 32). It is a time-consuming test and requires experience to read the slides.

Antinuclear antibodies (ANA or ANF)

Frozen sections of normal tissue (e.g. rat liver) are incubated with the patient's serum. The slide is then washed—leaving any antinuclear antibody adhering to the cell nuclei.

The next stage of this 'sandwich' technique is to incubate the section with goat antiserum to human gammaglobulin, the antiserum having first been conjugated to fluorescein. The fluorescinated antiserum adheres to the patient's serum wherever it is attached to the nuclei. After further washing the presence of antinuclear antibody can be detected by ultraviolet light microscopy as green fluorescence of nuclei. The pattern of staining varies (e.g. *see* p. 60). Results are reported as both titres and international units. The latter are standardised and therefore more reliable. Twenty-five iu/ml is significant. This corresponds to a titre of about 1/40, depending on the laboratory. More strongly positive tests correlate with more active disease.

This test is easy to perform, rapid and sensitive. It is positive in almost 100 per cent of patients with active SLE. It may also be positive in a variety of other disorders, including other connective tissue disease (p 32). It is a good screening test for SLE.

DNA antibody tests

Antibodies to native (double stranded) DNA are a relatively specific marker for SLE. They may be detected either by an immunochemical technique (*DNA-binding test*), or by an immunofluorescent method (*Crithidia luciliae test*).

DNA binding test. Radioactive (bacterial) double stranded DNA is mixed with the serum to be tested. The globulin fraction is then extracted, and its radioactivity measured to give an index of the DNA bound by antibody. Results over about 35 per cent (depending on the laboratory) are significant, and higher percentages generally reflect more active disease. The test is highly specific, but somewhat insensitive.

Crithidia luciliae test. This haemoflagellate possesses a giant mitochondrion containing double-stranded DNA. Using a sandwich technique (as in the fluorescent ANA test, p 133) it provides an alternative means of detecting antibodies to native DNA.

Antibodies to extractable nuclear antigens

Nuclei contain various 'extractable' (soluble) antigens. Autoantibodies to two of these have diagnostic significance. Both give a *speckled pattern* on fluorescent ANA testing (p 60). The one is an antibody to *nuclear ribonucleoprotein*. The other to a non-nucleic acid protein *Sm*. High titres of the former are characteristic of *mixed connective tissue disease*. Anti-Sm antibodies occur in SLE, not in mixed connective tissue disease.

Serum complement

When a 'complement fixing' antibody combines with its specific antigen it activates the cascade of complement enzymes. During this process the level of complement components in the serum falls as the individual factors are 'consumed' in the activation process. A fall in serum complement components is thus an indirect indication of the formation of circulating immune complexes. Such a fall is observed, for example, during active phases of systemic lupus erythematosus (p 37) and serum sickness (p 115). The most commonly employed measurements are *total haemolytic complement* (CH_{50}) and *C3*.

Antistreptolysin 'O' (ASO) titre

Haemolysin 'O' produced by streptococci is antigenic, and antibodies to it develop after a haemolytic streptococcal infection. The antibody is detected by its ability to inhibit haemolysis of sheep erythrocytes by streptolysin 'O'. A titre of 1/800 or a rising titre indicates a *recent streptococcal infection*. This is relevant when considering a diagnosis of rheumatic fever (p 99).

Synovial fluid examination

The main value of synovial fluid examination is to detect infection or identify crystals.

Appearance. Normal fluid is clear, straw-coloured, viscous and does not clot. Inflammatory changes are associated with larger volumes of cloudy fluid which is less viscous, and which clots on standing, due to the higher fibrinogen content.

Blood staining may indicate *trauma, haemophilia* (p 111) or *villo-nodular synovitis* (p 114). Septic arthritis characteristically produces a turbid fluid, but no reliance can be placed on the appearance.

Protein content. In degenerative joint disease the protein content is usually about 20 to 30 g/l. In inflammatory types of arthritis it may be 40 to 70 g/l. The rapid appearance of a firm clot indicates a high protein content.

Leucocytes. Synovial fluid for cell counts must immediately be mixed with EDTA anticoagulant, and acetic acid must be omitted from the diluting fluid. In osteoarthritis, leucocyte counts tend to be below 1×10^9/l; in rheumatoid arthritis they are usually over 3×10^9/l (sometimes much higher), but there is a very wide overlap. The percentage of polymorphonuclear leucocytes is also highly variable. It tends to be below 50 per cent in osteoarthritis, greater than 50 per cent in rheumatoid arthritis, and over 95 per cent in septic arthritis.

Microbiology. Microbiological examination of synovial fluid follows conventional lines. It goes without saying that, in suspected septic arthritis, it is critical to obtain both synovial fluid and blood for microbiological examination before antibiotics are started.

Crystals in synovial fluid. Fluid for crystal examination is taken without anticoagulant. Any clot that forms will enmesh crystals, and it is thus essential to examine a piece of the clot. Crystals of both *urate* (p 79) and *pyrophosphate* (p 88) are birefringent and thus easily detected by *polarised light microscopy*. Further, their different optical properties allow them to be differentiated with confidence.

Synovial biopsy

Specimens of synovium for histology may be obtained either by *open arthrotomy* or by *closed needle biopsy*. Indications include cases of monarticular arthritis in which tuberculosis is a possibility.

Arthroscopy

Continuing technical advances in endoscopic equipment are making arthroscopy a very simple and safe procedure under local or general anaesthesia. This technique finds its main usefulness in the knee: assessing the state of the menisci, seeking loose bodies, and investigating the cause of unexplained knee joint pain.

Thermography

Skin temperature reflects vascularity, and can be documented as an *infrared-thermographic 'map'* of a joint. This provides an objective, albeit elaborate, technique for recording one aspect of inflammation. It has not yet found a useful place in routine practice.

Radio-isotopic scanning

Radioactivity over a joint can be measured or recorded as an image following a relatively harmless intravenous dose of *technetium-99m*. This reflects blood flow. Linking the isotope to a 'bone seeking' chemical, for example methylene diphosphoric acid (MDP) provides a means of detecting areas of increased bone turnover. Radioactive bone imaging provides an extremely valuable means of seeking secondary malignant deposits or infections in bone, particularly in the spine. However, its usefulness in the diagnosis of arthritis is less clear. It provides, like thermography (*see above*) a somewhat elaborate, but objective, means of recording articular blood flow. It is of value in detecting early evidence of aseptic necrosis (p 109), and it is being tested as a method of identifying early sacroilitis.

Index

Systemic sclerosis, 39–43
  aetiology, 39
  clinical features, 39
  course and prognosis, 42
  CRST (CREST) syndrome, 40
  laboratory findings, 41
  pathology, 39
  Sjögren's syndrome, 41
  Thibierge-Weissenbach syndrome,
    40
  treatment, 42

Takayasu's arteritis, 49
Technetium scan, 136
Telangiectasia in systemic sclerosis,
    40
Temporal arteritis, 45–7 (*see also*
    Giant cell arteritis)
Temporal artery biopsy
  in giant cell arteritis, 46
  in polymyalgia rheumatica, 48
Temporomandibular joint,
    examination of, 126
Tenderness, joint, 123
Tendinitis, 101 (*see also* Shoulder
    joint *and* Tenosynovitis)
  Achilles', 22, 23, 106
  biceps, 103
  calcific, 102
  supraspinatus, 102
Tennis elbow, 104
Tenosynovitis
  de Quervain's, 106
  in gonococcal infections, 93
  in rheumatoid arthritis, 4, 7
  in Reiter's disease, 30
  in systemic sclerosis, 41
  trigger finger, 7, 106, 118
Thermography, 136
Thibierge-Weissenbach syndrome,
    40
Thoracic duct drainage, 38
Thoraco-lumbar spine, examination
    of, 125
Thrombocytopenia
  in Felty's syndrome, 8
  in Sjögren's syndrome, 58
  in systemic lupus erythematosus,
    36
Tinel's sign, 105

Toes, examination of, 131
Torticollis, 71
Trabecular fractures in
    osteoarthritis, 62
Traction
  cervical, 71, 73
  lumbar, 75
Transfusion siderosis, 111
Trendelenberg test, 52, 128
Trigeminal nerve lesions in systemic
    sclerosis, 41
Trigger finger, 7, 106, 118
Tuberculous arthritis, 94–5
Tumours, synovial, 116

Ulceration
  buccal
    in Behçet's syndrome, 109
    in Reiter's disease, 30
  genital, in Behçet's syndrome, 109
  skin
    in Behçet's syndrome, 109
    in Felty's syndrome, 8
    in rheumatoid arthritis, 7
Ulcerative colitis, 21, 31
Ulnar deviation of fingers in
    rheumatoid arthritis, 6
Ulnar nerve compression, 105
Urate, *see* Uric acid
Urethritis, 29
Uric acid (and urate), 79
  calculi, 82
  deposition in tissues, 81
  excretion, 81
  identification of crystals, 135
  metabolism, 79
  plasma levels, 81
    effect of dietary purines, 81
    in psoriasis, 27
  renal handling, 81
    factors modifying, 81
Uricase, 79
Uricosuric drugs, 81, 86
Urolithiasis (urate), 82
Uveitis
  in ankylosing spondylitis, 21, 26
  in Behçet's syndrome, 109
  in juvenile chronic arthritis, 15,
    16
  in Reiter's disease, 30